TALLER THAN A TREE

Copyright Abraham Thomas 2024

All rights reserved. No part of the contents of this book may be reproduced in any manner whatsoever without written permission, except in the case of brief descriptions and critical articles.

First Printing 2024.

ABRAHAM THOMAS

TALLER THAN A TREE

THE XCODE MIND

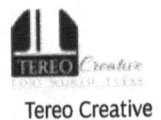

Tereo Creative

Abraham Thomas, a mechanical engineering graduate from Guindy and a production engineering post-graduate from Imperial College, London, brings a unique blend of technical expertise and real-world experience to his writing. His diverse background as a manufacturer of electrical equipment and a builder informs his insightful exploration of the developmental effects of urbanization in his book, *The Affluence Machine*. Delving into the complexities of human cognition, Thomas's writings also propose that intelligence may arise from neural pattern recognition and delve into the emotional nuances triggered by intuition.

TO
SARASU, BIJU AND SARA
WHO MADE THIS BOOK POSSIBLE

CONTENTS

1 — THE AMBITIOUS DREAM OF SIGMUND FREUD
1

2 — THE CURIOUS CASE OF ELIMINATION
5

3 — THE xCode
8

4 — THE TRIUNE BRAIN
14

5 — INTUITIVE DECISION MAKING
21

6 — MEMORIES IN TRANSPLANTED ORGANS
25

7 — THE UNCONSCIOUS THOUGHT THEORY
29

8 — THE AMYGDALA
32

CONTENTS

9 — SENSORY RECEPTORS
36

10 — A THEORY OF HUMOR
39

11 — DETERMINISM VS FREE WILL
43

12 — DEFINE COMMON SENSE
47

13 — HUMAN MEMORY RESEARCH MISTAKE
52

14 — HUMAN MEMORY CAPACITY
56

15 — THE INSULAR CORTEX
59

16 — MIRROR NEURONS
64

17 — THE SOCIAL COMPARISON THEORY
68

18 — LONG TERM POTENTIATION
73

19 — BEHAVIOR PATTERN RECOGNITION
76

CONTENTS

20 — THE ORIENTING RESPONSE
80

21 — THE SOMATIC MARKER HYPOTHESIS
84

22 — THE SAVANT BRAIN
88

23 — THE MEANING OF CONSCIOUSNESS
92

24 — WHERE DO THOUGHTS COME FROM?
96

25 — WHAT IS A BELIEF?
100

26 — WHAT IS KNOWLEDGE?
104

27 — WORKING MEMORY
108

28 — WHAT CAUSES EMOTIONS
112

29 — A COSMIC INTELLIGENCE
116

30 — MIND CONTROL TIPS
120

PREFACE

A tree stands tall and proud, its roots firmly planted in the earth. It grows, it changes, it adapts to its environment. But it is bound by its biology, by the unyielding laws of nature. It cannot uproot itself and seek a new home, nor can it ponder the mysteries of the universe or create a symphony.

You, on the other hand, are taller than a tree.

You may think intelligence is the ability to acquire and apply knowledge, solve problems, and adapt to new situations. And you'd be right – to a point. Philosophers, psychologists, and cognitive scientists have studied and debated this complex trait for centuries, proposing various models and theories to understand and measure its many facets.

But what if intelligence isn't just about *what* we think, but *how* we think? What if there's a fundamental biological mechanism that underlies all our cognitive abilities, a spark that ignites the process of uncovering the unknown?

PREFACE

A spark that separates us from the rooted existence of trees?

This book delves into a groundbreaking theory that sheds light on the biological underpinnings of our intelligent minds. Instead of focusing on the impact of intelligence, we uncover a previously overlooked neurological phenomenon – xCode – which serves as the starting point of intelligence itself: the process of discovering the "x," the unknown. This process not only elucidates how we think but also explains why we sometimes act in ways that are profoundly illogical or counterproductive.

Through vivid anecdotes and clarifying scientific explanations, we embark on a mind-expanding journey to understand how this remarkable biological phenomenon manifests in the intelligent behaviors we see in humans, animals, and even our latest AI creations. From the inexplicable flashes of insight that solve complex problems, to the baffling lapses in judgment that leave us scratching our heads, xCode sheds new light on the full spectrum of human intelligence.

Along the way, we explore cutting-edge research on the different brain regions and neurochemical processes that contribute to our cognitive capabilities. Discover how our emotions, beliefs, and even our sense of humor are inextricably linked to this foundational aspect of our neurobiology.

PREFACE

As you delve deeper, you'll be left in awe of the elegant, yet often counterintuitive, ways our brains generate intelligent behavior. And you'll be left to ponder the profound implications – both exciting and unsettling – of unlocking the biological code of human intelligence. Where will this knowledge lead us as we continue to push the boundaries of artificial intelligence? The answers may surprise you.

Prepare to have your understanding of your own mind revolutionized. This is science writing at its most engaging and enlightening, opening up new frontiers of knowledge that will forever change how you think about thinking. And it will help you understand why you, with your extraordinary xCode, cast a longer shadow than a tree.

THE AMBITIOUS DREAM OF SIGMUND FREUD

It was a time of great change and turmoil in the late 19th century. The rapid advancements in science and technology had shaken the very foundations of how people understood the world. Nowhere was this more true than in the realm of the human mind - that mysterious black box that governed our thoughts, emotions, and behaviors.

Into this intellectual maelstrom stepped an ambitious young Viennese physician named Sigmund Freud. Freud was determined to crack the code of the human psyche, to peer into the darkness of the unconscious and uncover its deepest secrets. Like an explorer venturing into uncharted territory, he set out to map the uncharted landscape of the mind.

Freud's approach was both revolutionary and controversial. Inspired by his mentor Josef Breuer's work with "talking cures", Freud developed a new therapeutic method he called psychoanalysis. The idea was deceptively simple - by guiding patients to uncover and confront their repressed thoughts and memories, Freud believed he could liberate them from the shackles of the unconscious and cure their neuroses.

At the heart of Freud's theory was a tripartite model of the mind - the id, the ego, and the superego. The id, Freud proposed, represented our most primal, animal-like instincts - the raw drives for sex, aggression, and pleasure. The ego was the rational, problem-solving part of the mind that mediated between the id's demands and the constraints of the external world. And the superego was the internalized voice of moral conscience, scolding us when we strayed from societal norms.

Like a three-way tug-of-war, Freud saw the psyche as the battleground where these three forces constantly vied for dominance. Neuroses and mental disorders, he believed, were the result of imbalances and conflicts between the id, ego, and superego.

It was a grand, sweeping theory - an ambitious attempt to map the hidden topography of the human mind. And for a time, Freud's ideas captivated the public imagination. Psychoanalysis became all the rage, with Freudian analysts setting up shop in major cities around the world. His theories on sexuality, the Oedipus complex, and dream interpretation captivated the intellectual zeitgeist.

But Freud's tripartite model of the mind was not without its critics. Many psychologists and neuroscientists questioned the lack of empirical evidence supporting his theories. They argued that Freud had built his edifice of psychoanalysis on the shaky foundation of anecdotal data, dream analysis, and free association techniques.

As our scientific understanding of the brain and human behavior has evolved, many of Freud's core ideas have been challenged or debunked. The simplistic divisions of the id, ego, and superego now seem like an overly reductive view of the dazzlingly complex workings of the human mind.

Yet, for all its flaws, Freud's ambitious dream of cracking the code of the unconscious left an indelible mark on our culture. His insights into the power of the subconscious, the role of sexuality in human development, and the importance of early childhood experiences continue to reverberate today. Freud may not have discovered the secrets of the mind, but he set in motion a revolution in how we understand ourselves.\

In the end, Freud's legacy is a cautionary tale - a reminder that even the grandest of theories must constantly be tested, refined, and updated in the face of new evidence. The journey to understanding intelligence is a never-ending one, filled with both breakthroughs and blind alleys. But Freud's courageous attempt to illuminate the mysterious workings of the mind will always be remembered as a crucial first step on that long, winding path.

THE CURIOUS CASE OF ELIMINATION

Can a humble spreadsheet experiment yield a profound revelation about the nature of intelligence itself? Your initial goal was a familiar one – to create an "expert system" capable of diagnosing diseases based on symptoms, emulating the decision-making process of an experienced physician. However, the traditional approach of encoding complex branching logic and exhaustive "if-then" rules soon revealed its limitations.

It was then that a simple spreadsheet revealed the drama of an elegant alternative approach. You input 10 diseases and 33 potential symptoms, initially including all possibilities. But instead of having the system laboriously follow a predetermined decision tree, you took a simple, but contrary route – one by one, you started deleting all the diseases that didn't match each indicated symptom.

The results were striking. With each deletion, the spreadsheet rapidly narrowed down the options. Often it pinpointed the correct diagnosis with just a single, definitive symptom. It was a dramatic parallel to how a seasoned doctor might swiftly eliminate multiple potential diagnoses with just a cursory glance, cutting through the noise to focus on the essential patterns.

This simple yet profound experiment shed light on a compelling possibility concerning human intelligence. Unlike an orthodox expert system, blindly plodding through checklists of rules, the mind could be eliminating vast swaths of irrelevant information to leap to a single pattern leading to the solution. But, the information had to exist in the mind before it could be eliminated. Could all that data be stored as memories?

There was no clear theory about how the mind stored memories. You only knew that the mind could remember trillions of images. But, intuition could be the mechanism that facilitates the brain's ability to sift through an astronomical amount of stored knowledge and intuitively leap to conclusions by instantly recognizing patterns and discarding what doesn't fit. It challenged the traditional notion that intelligence is solely defined by IQ scores, academic achievements, or the ability to rigidly follow predetermined rules.

Your spreadsheet experiment highlighted the possibility that the mind could transcend the limitations of rigid algorithms and expert systems to seamlessly integrate vast amounts of information, recognize salient patterns by swiftly discarding irrelevant data.

The possibility that the mind was recognizing patterns could reshape our understanding of human cognition, problem-solving, and decision-making processes. It could open new avenues for exploration in fields as diverse as cognitive science, artificial intelligence, and education, challenging us to rethink how we nurture and cultivate intelligence in all its multifaceted forms.

The humble spreadsheet may have sparked a revolution in our comprehension of the mind's remarkable abilities, reminding us that true intelligence often lies not in the strict adherence to rules, but in the adaptive, intuitive capacity to recognize patterns and eliminate irrelevance – a quality that sets the human mind apart as a truly remarkable problem-solving machine.

THE XCODE

Introduction

At the heart of our incredible capacity for intelligence lies a powerful mechanism within the fundamental units of our brain - the neurons. The XCode proposes that neurons employ immense memory storage to precisely match and integrate a multitude of factors before triggering signals that underlie our thoughts, emotions, and even consciousness itself.

In the tightly packed 20-micron spaces of living cells, DNA provides the blueprints while dynamic epigenetic changes add layers of memory and adaptation. Similarly, the XCode hypothesis suggests that neurons have staggering memory capacities that allow them to match combinatorial patterns of incoming signals against a complex tapestry of genetic instructions, protein memories, subthreshold potentials, and neurochemical signatures.

The Vast Scale of Neuronal Processing

To grasp the incredible scale of information processing implied by the XCode, we need only consider one of the many factors neurons routinely integrate - the combinatorial coding required to recognize trillions of distinct odors. The sheer memory storage and computational power required for such exquisite odor discrimination is staggering, yet this represents just a minuscule fraction of what neurons accomplish.

Indeed, the XCode points to neurons as being sophisticated molecular computers, with astronomically large memory banks allowing them to precisely match a wide array of multi-modal data from across the brain and body. This paints a profound new picture of single neurons as dynamic information processing hubs rather than simple relays.

The Factors Enabling Disinhibition

So how exactly do individual neurons integrate all this rich multi-modal information from myriad sources to trigger precise, contextualized disinhibition signals? Let's delve into five key factors the XCode proposes neurons can match:

1. Combinatorial Patterns of Incoming Links

A neuron doesn't just receive random input - it receives

information from very specific groups of other neurons connected via intricate patterns of synaptic links. Just like a password, a unique arrangement and sequence of activation across these many incoming connections from an ensemble of associated neurons may be required to trigger disinhibition in the target cell.

2. Genetic Information

Far from being generic information transmitters, a neuron's genetic underpinnings essentially code its unique identity and information processing role. The specific genetic makeup of a neuron dictates the type of neurotransmitter receptors it will express, determining the neurotransmitters it can respond to. Genetics also guides the formation of very precise connection patterns during development, allowing for the targeted delivery of inhibition. Even at a micro-circuit level, like those involved in visual edge detection, genetics can fine-tune the arrangement and function of excitatory and inhibitory neuron types.

3. Protein Memories

Neurons are not passive receivers of information - they are constantly adapting by modifying the very physical structures and molecular machinery within them based on experiences and activity patterns. Changes in protein structures, such as those underlying long-term potentiation of synapses, act as physical memories that shape how a neuron will respond to future input patterns. These rich protein memories contribute to the overall pattern recognition and processing capabilities of individual neurons.

4. Subthreshold Potentials

Not all incoming signals have sufficient strength to trigger full-blown action potentials to be transmitted down a neuron's axon. However, these subthreshold signals from various sources can summate, with their collective effect contributing to whether the neuron reaches the threshold to trigger disinhibition. By exquisitely integrating these subthreshold "details", neurons can build a high-resolution picture of the total input pattern before deciding whether to propagate a signal.

5. Neurochemical Signatures

The information represented by patterns of neurotransmitters released into the extracellular environment surrounding a neuron creates a distinct neurochemical signature in the synaptic clefts along its surface. This dynamic neurochemical "bath" that the neuron is immersed in can significantly influence its excitability, the degree to which it is inhibited or disinhibited, and the nature of the signals it transmits or receives.

The Implications

By seamlessly integrating such a wide breadth of multidimensional data points - precise synaptic connectivity patterns, genetic programming, molecular records of past activity, subthreshold signals, and the neuron's biochemical context - the XCode proposes that individual neurons can match the total input against astronomically large memory capacities. This allows them to trigger precise disinhibition signals at the axon hillock only when the most relevant and specific conditions are met.

The implications of such staggeringly complex, dynamic, context-aware molecular information processing within our neurons are profound. It suggests that cognitive phenomena like conscious awareness, emotions, decision-making and more arise not just from connections between neurons, but from these tiny cellular reactors performing high-dimensional calculus limited only by the immense memory and computational capacities available at the molecular scale.

The XCode truly represents a profound rethinking of the neuron itself - not as a simple relay, but as an incredibly sophisticated molecular computer blending memories, genetics, biochemical signals and more into a unified high-resolution representation that allows precise and context-specific control of disinhibition signals out to the rest of the brain and body.

In the chapters ahead, we'll explore how the core principles of the XCode illuminate our understanding of sensory perception, cognition, learning, consciousness, and the very nature of intelligence. But first, we must set the stage by diving deeper into the emerging evidence for each of the key factors the XCode proposes neurons integrate to enable this pivotal process of targeted disinhibition at the axon hillock.

CHAPTER 4

THE TRIUNE BRAIN

My friends, have you ever felt like there's a constant tug-of-war raging inside your head? As if the rational, analytical part of your brain is at odds with some deeper, primal force - an animal voice that seems to have a mind of its own? Well, you're not alone. In fact, this mental tussle is a direct consequence of the incredible evolutionary journey that shaped the human mind into the marvel it is today.

You see, our brains didn't emerge fully formed in one fell swoop. No, they are an architectural masterpiece constructed layer by layer over millions of years of evolution. Imagine your mind as an ancient cathedral, built up one stunning level at a time. At the base, we have the reptilian brain - the oldest, most primitive part that deals with our most basic survival instincts and drives. This is the security guard of the cathedral, always on high alert, ready to sound alarms or lash out aggressively at the slightest perceived threat.

But our evolution didn't stop there. Surrounding this reptilian core, we developed the mammalian brain - the emotional center that lets us experience the full kaleidoscope of feelings, from the blissful comfort of a mother's embrace to the searing sting of heartbreak. Picture this as the cathedral's stained glass windows, casting a warm glow of vibrant emotions over the entire structure. It's the gut-level intuitive voice that can sometimes override our rational thinking in the heat of the moment.

Finally, perched atop these ancient foundations like towering spires reaching for the heavens, we have the prefrontal cortex regions - the pinnacle of our brain's evolution. This is the seat of our higher cognitive abilities like reasoning, judgment, and willpower. It's the part that might advise you that giving in to your furious anger or consuming desires is probably unwise, even as your emotional brain is screaming at you to act.

The triune brain theory that so elegantly explains the conflicting forces that shape our intuitions didn't simply appear out of the ether. No, it was the brilliant work of a pioneering neuroscientist named Paul D. MacLean who first mapped out this revolutionary model of the human mind.

MacLean was a true visionary, a scientist with a storyteller's gift for looking at the brain through an evolutionary lens. In the 1960s, he proposed that the human mind emerged not as a single unified system, but rather as a successive layering of three distinct "brains" over the long ancestral march of evolution.

Drawing on decades of anatomical and behavioral research, MacLean theorized that we humans are essentially sculpted atop the evolutionary foundations laid by our distant reptilian and mammalian forebears. The reptilian brain formed first as a primordial knot of structures governing basic arousal, aggression, dominance, and rituals related to territory and mating. It was the original "", operating primarily on instinct and reflex.

Then came the arrival of early mammalian species, whose environmental pressures selected for the emergence of a powerful new brain layer surrounding that reptilian core. This was the limbic system - a hodgepodge of intricate structures like the amygdala, hippocampus, and cingulate cortex that gave rise to the vast new realms of emotion, memory, and social behavior that we warm-blooded mammals experienced.

Finally, millions of years later, the upright primates and then early humans evolved the massive prefrontal cortex that forms the headier, more conscious and rational outer layers of the modern brain. This prefrontal "CEO" gave us the ability for abstract reasoning, willful decision-making, long-term planning, and other hallmarks of intelligence as we know it.

But here's the crucial point that MacLean realized - these three successive brain "formations" didn't simply replace one another in a linear progression. Rather, they accumulated atop the previous layers, coexisting in an obligatory relationship of constant interplay and potential conflict. The primitive reptilian impulses were still there, doing battle with the emotional drives and intuitions of the mammalian brain, which were in turn superseded and moderated by the prefrontal executive regions.

It was this triune constellation of interacting systems, proposed MacLean, that shaped our mental experience into the complex, chaotic symphony of logical analysis, gut feelings, and primal urges that we know so well. The turf wars between these three semi-independent "brains" sculpted the landscape of human behavior, producing both the creative flashes of intuitive brilliance and the bouts of irrational, self-sabotaging folly that define our species.

MacLean's vision revealed the secrets of the triune brain in a way that was as insightful as it was poetic. By looking at the human mind through the lens of our ancestral past, he uncovered the mystery of how we became the gloriously irrational, intuitive, intelligent creatures we are today. His ideas forever changed how we think about thinking itself.

Now here's where things get really intriguing. You see, this triune structure means that the human mind is essentially run by three quasi-independent "brains" locked in an eternal dance of cooperation and conflict. Our primitive reptilian urges butt heads with our mammalian emotional drives, while our prefrontal regions try to play the rational referee.

And this dynamic interplay is the heart of our intuitive experience. You know that flash of insight, that sudden "aha!" moment when the solution to a vexing problem just seems to pop into your conscious mind? That's your intuition speaking up - a direct product of the brilliance and loopy irrationality of the XCode mechanism hard at work.

Through its uncanny pattern recognition abilities, XCode scans the inputs from your senses and memories, looking for matches to the patterns encoded in your neurons over a lifetime of experiences. When it detects a familiar combination, it disinhibits and activates the corresponding neuron cluster, allowing their collective wisdom to bubble up into your conscious awareness as an intuitive hunch or flash of insight.

But XCode doesn't just conjure intuitions from thin air - it's heavily influenced by the whims and agendas of your triune brain layers. You see, when your emotional brain is in the grip of a powerful feeling like fear, anger or desire, XCode automatically biases its scanning to align with that state. It suppresses any patterns that might conflict with your current emotional perspective while amplifying any information that supports and justifies how you're feeling in the moment.

It's like a filter that tints your intuitive insights with the prevailing emotional overtones. When you're furious at a romantic partner, for instance, XCode will preferentially highlight any memories or patterns that feed your feelings of betrayal and righteous indignation while shutting out any mitigating evidence. Your intuition becomes a funhouse mirror, reflecting back your own distorted emotional reality.

This dynamic is one key reason our intuitions can sometimes lead us so disastrously astray - because they emerge from the irrational undercurrents of our triune minds rather than from pure, impartial logic. Your intuitive flashes of insight are the product of an ancient, evolved mechanism that is inherently biased and shaped by your primal urges and turbulent feelings.

But that's not to say intuition is inherently bad or something to be ignored. Like any human faculty, it has both strengths and weaknesses that stem from the quirks of its underlying biology and evolution. The key is to understand where your intuitions come from and how they can be warped by the undercurrents of your triune mind's interplay.

When you can step back and recognize that your intuitive inklings are colored by the whims of your emotional brain or reptilian impulses, you'll be much better equipped to test those intuitions against logic and evidence. You can use the rational prowess of your prefrontal cortex to scrutinize and refine your intuitive hunches rather than blindly following wherever your biased intuitions lead.

In this way, intuition can be an incredibly powerful adjunct to analysis and conscious reasoning rather than a capricious master to be obeyed. By understanding the triune structure of your mind and the secrets of XCode, you can learn to take advantage of intuition's insights while remaining grounded in rationality and open-mindedness.

So the next time you feel that little voice pipe up with a powerful conviction or flash of insight, don't immediately heed its siren song. Stop, listen to your intuition's whispers, but then engage your prefrontal regions to logically evaluate whether this intuitive feeling stands up to scrutiny. Leverage the full power of your triune mind rather than letting any one part dominate. With this balanced approach, my friends, you'll be infinitely better poised to navigate the complexities of life with wisdom and clarity.

INTUITIVE DECISION MAKING

Have you ever found yourself faced with a difficult decision, hesitating for what feels like an eternity, only to suddenly have a "eureka" moment and spring into action? That, my friends, is the power of intuitive decision-making - a remarkable feat of the human mind that has captivated thinkers and scientists for centuries.

Join Thomas as we delve into the intricate workings of this mental marvel, guided by the insightful observations of none other than the legendary William James. Imagine, if you will, a young lad snuggled up in the cozy warmth of his bed, reluctant to face the bitter chill of a winter morning. As James so eloquently described, the "cozy warmth under the blanket" battles with the "shivering cold signaling the day's drudgery." The lad lies there, unable to muster the willpower to get up.

But then, something remarkable happens. A "lucky idea" suddenly awakens, one that "awakens no contradictory or paralyzing suggestions." Boom! Just like that, the negative feelings are stilled, and the young man springs into action, leaving the comfort of his bed behind. James called this a shift from "wish" to an act of "will" - a testament to the astonishing power of our intuitive decision-making.

But how, you ask, does this mysterious process unfold within the confines of our minds? Well, my friends, it's a fascinating tale of a veritable United Nations of intelligences, all vying for control like a zany political circus. Imagine your brain as a country, with a triune government made up of the mighty reptilian, mammalian, and prefrontal regions, each with its own agenda and decision-making hierarchy.

At the lowest levels, we have the individual "actors" - the neurons and their interconnected networks, making their own decisions like a bunch of mischievous city council members. As we climb the political ladder, the "communities" of the limbic system and spinal cord take the reins, orchestrating a complex dance of emotions, sensations, and muscle movements. And finally, at the top, we have the "central government" of the prefrontal regions, where the real "you" resides, wielding the power of reason and logic (or at least, trying to).

But here's the kicker: your trusty prefrontal regions may think they're in charge, but more often than not, the emotional overlords of the limbic system are the ones pulling the strings. Like a crafty politician, your emotions can overrule your best intentions faster than it takes for spilled coffee to hit the saucer. That's when you quit admiring the problem.

Imagine, for a moment, that you're in an elevator, and the sudden urge to raise your arms strikes you. "No problem," you think, "I'll just use my mighty will to make it happen." But alas, the moment you try, your mind's internal security forces (a.k.a. the WASP - Worthwhile, Appropriate, Safe, and Practical considerations) swoop in and shut down your plan faster than lightning.

So, if your will isn't always the ultimate decision-maker, what is? Well, my friends, it's the intricate dance of that million-fibered limbic system, with its feedback and feedforward links, that ultimately calls the shots. Just like the spinal cord's masterful coordination of muscle contractions, the limbic system is a virtuoso at managing the complex interplay of our emotions, guiding us through the twists and turns of everyday life.

Thomas explains that it has adapted the same logic underlying the smooth, fluid movements of our motor systems, using XCode. Just as motor neurons coordinate muscle contractions, the limbic system leverages XCode to match incoming information against a vast library of stored emotional memories, triggering precise patterns of inhibition and expression. It's this intricate, near-instantaneous process that allows our limbic system to exert such profound influence over our thoughts, decisions, and sense of self - all while our conscious, "rational" minds remain blissfully unaware of the hidden neural drama unfolding beneath the surface.

And the beauty of it all is that this remarkable system is the product of eons of evolutionary adaptation. As the brilliant Francois Jacob so eloquently observed, "evolution does not produce innovations from scratch. It works on what already exists, either transforming a system to give it a new function or combining several systems to produce a more complex one." In other words, our intuitive decision-making is the culmination of nature's innovation of the spinal cord, a testament to the sheer genius of evolution.

So, the next time you find yourself in the throes of a tough decision, take a moment to appreciate the incredible journey your mind is about to embark on. Who knows, you might just surprise yourself as you spring into action, leaving that cozy bed behind and embracing the day ahead. The mind's a marvel, isn't it?

CHAPTER 6

MEMORIES IN TRANSPLANTED ORGANS

Claire's story makes one feel a sense of wonder and disbelief. This unassuming woman had undergone a heart transplant, and the changes in her personality and behavior were nothing short of remarkable.

According to the research outlined in the paper, numerous organ transplant recipients have reported acquiring the memories, experiences, and even emotions of their deceased donors. This phenomenon points to the possibility that our major organs, like the heart, may possess their own form of "cellular memory." (All about XCode)

Take the case of the eight-year-old girl who received the heart of a murdered ten-year-old. After the surgery, the young recipient began having vivid, recurring nightmares about the murder. When questioned by the police, she provided shockingly accurate details about the crime - "the time, the weapon, the place, the clothes he wore, what the little girl he killed had said to him... everything the little heart transplant recipient reported was completely accurate."

Or consider the story of Claire Sylvia herself. After receiving a heart transplant, Sylvia reported acquiring her donor's love for chicken nuggets, green peppers, and beer. She even found herself dressing in cooler colors, abandoning the bright reds and oranges she used to favor. Sylvia's personality took on a more aggressive, impulsive edge as well, mirroring that of her anonymous donor.

"It was as if I had been imbued with a whole new set of memories, preferences, and tendencies that weren't my own," Sylvia later wrote in her book, A Change of Heart.

These are not isolated incidents. Another heart transplant recipient, a middle-aged Caucasian man, reportedly developed a taste for classical music - the same passion his African-American teenage donor had been known for. And William Sheridan, a retired catering manager with poor drawing skills, suddenly blossomed into an accomplished artist after his transplant surgery, discovering his donor had been a keen painter.

"It's as if the transplanted organ isn't just a physical replacement, but a carrier of emotional and behavioral DNA," explained Dr. Andrew Armour, a pioneer in the field of neurocardiology. "The heart, in particular, seems to possess this remarkable capacity to store combinatorial memories and influence our very sense of self." (Not just the heart, all the 86 billion neurons).

The implications of this phenomenon are truly astounding. Our organs may not be the passive vessels we've long assumed, but rather complex, interconnected systems capable of influencing our thoughts, feelings, and behaviors in profound ways.

At the heart of this capability lies the XCode - a hypothesis that explains how neurons are able to match incoming information against a vast library of stored memories, triggering precise patterns of disinhibition at the axon hillock. These neurological processes underlie our intuition, emotions, intelligence, and even consciousness itself.

Within the 20-micron confines of each of our 86 billion neurons, a virtually infinite array of memory factors are encoded and are constantly being matched against incoming signals at the trillions of synapses throughout our bodies, in a complex combinatorial dance akin to how our sense of smell recognizes countless combinations of odors.

It is this intricate, near-instantaneous pattern matching that allows our organs, like the heart, to exert such a profound influence on our thoughts, feelings, and behaviors. We're not just walking around with a physical replacement organ - we're carrying with us the unique memories, experiences, and even personalities of our donors, encoded in the very rhythms of our heartbeats.

The more you learn about these cases of cellular memory in organ transplants, the more you marveled at the hidden depths of the human body. Who knows what other secrets our organs might be keeping, just waiting to be unlocked? It's enough to make you wonder if you're truly the master of your own mind, or if there's a whole symphony playing beneath the surface, orchestrated by the subtle rhythms of your very own heart - a veritable "brain" in its own right, processing a lifetime of memories and experiences.

CHAPTER
7

THE UNCONSCIOUS THOUGHT THEORY

Have you ever had one of those fleeting moments of brilliance, where the solution to a problem just seemed to pop into your head, unbidden? Or found yourself drawn to certain people, places, or activities, with no clear rational explanation? If so, you may have been experiencing the workings of a remarkable cognitive phenomenon described by Thomas as the Intuitive Unconscious Thought Theory (IUTT).

The IUTT proposes that the vast majority of our thought processes - the ones that enable us to make sense of the world, set goals, and make predictions - happen entirely outside the realm of our conscious awareness. Our conscious mind, it seems, is merely the tip of the iceberg, a narrow mirror reflecting the outcomes of a grand, unseen symphony orchestrated by what IUTT calls the "blind watchmaker" of our unconscious.

This notion may seem counterintuitive at first. Aren't we the masters of our own minds, guiding our thoughts and actions through sheer willpower? Not according to the IUTT. Groundbreaking research by scientists like Benjamin Libet has already shown that our brains often make decisions long before we're consciously aware of them.

In one of Libet's experiments, participants were asked to press a button while monitoring a constantly shifting dot on a screen. The participants reported the precise moment they consciously decided to press the button. But Libet's measurements revealed that their brain had actually triggered the motor activity to press the button a full 350 milliseconds before the "conscious decision" was made.

"So you're telling me that the little voice in my head that thinks it's in charge is actually just a passenger on the train?" You ask with a bemused chuckle. Thomas replies "Exactly. The real decision-making is happening in the unconscious realms of the mind - what IUTT calls the 'blind watchmaker.' Our conscious awareness is just along for the ride, observing the outcomes rather than controlling the process."

Our neurons are constantly comparing the information they receive against an almost unimaginable database of past experiences and knowledge. We've all got a 'blind genius' inside our heads, working tirelessly to make sense of the world around us. Who knows what other remarkable feats our unconscious thought processes might be capable of, if only we could peer behind the veil of conscious awareness?

One thing's for certain: the next time you find yourself struck by a sudden flash of insight or an inexplicable gut feeling, take a moment to appreciate the intricate dance of neurological activity happening within the hidden recesses of your brain. Because the true genius of the human mind lies not in the spotlight of consciousness, but in the symphony of the unseen.

CHAPTER 8

THE AMYGDALA

Have you ever found yourself reacting to a situation with an intense surge of emotion - anger, fear, or even gut-wrenching grief - before you even had a chance to consciously process what was happening? Well, my friends, you can thank a tiny, almond-shaped structure deep within your brain for that: the amygdala.

The amygdala is one of the unsung heroes of our central nervous system, working tirelessly behind the scenes to protect us from harm. You see, these small nuclei are responsible for interpreting subtle, subconscious cues of danger or threat, and triggering lightning-fast responses to keep us safe. It's like having a tenacious bouncer at the door of your mind, always on the lookout for potential troublemakers.

Now, you might be thinking, "But wait, I thought the brain was all about cool, rational thinking! What's this emotional cowboy doing in there?" Well, the truth is, the amygdala is a crucial part of the limbic system - the ancient, primal region of the brain that governs our feelings and instincts. And it's been protecting our ancestors since the dawn of time.

You see, back in the good old days when saber-toothed tigers were still a thing, the amygdala was the first line of defense against mortal danger. Its pattern recognition circuits could detect the faintest whiff of a threat, triggering a burst of adrenaline and preparing the body to fight, flee, or freeze. It was a matter of life and death, and the amygdala was the gatekeeper that kept us alive.

But the amygdala's influence extends far beyond just physical threats. As our brains evolved, these emotional powerhouses also became attuned to the more nuanced social cues that governed herd life. They learned to recognize the subtle signs of anger, fear, or disgust on the faces of our fellow primates, allowing us to navigate the complex web of relationships and avoid potential conflict.

In fact, research has shown that the amygdala is so sensitive to these social signals that it can even detect them in the faces of complete strangers. It's like the amygdala has a sixth sense for picking up on negative vibes - a handy skill, to be sure, but one that can sometimes lead to over-reactions and knee-jerk responses that make us do, well, some pretty "stupid" things.

The amygdala is like a sensitive smoke alarm - it goes off at the first whiff of trouble, even if it's just a little toast burning in the toaster.

But the amygdala's role in our emotional lives doesn't stop there. These powerhouses of the brain are also responsible for forming and storing memories of traumatic or intensely emotional experiences. Through a process called "long-term potentiation," the amygdala can hold onto the neural patterns associated with past stressful events, triggering those familiar feelings of fear, anger, or grief at the slightest provocation.

It's like the amygdala has a secret vault of emotional souvenirs, each one waiting to be dusted off and thrust back into the spotlight at the most inopportune moments. The amygdala is like a grumpy old man with a long memory - it never forgets a slight, and it's always ready to give you an earful about it.

Fortunately, our brains are a lot more sophisticated than we give them credit for. While the amygdala may be the emotional powerhouse, it's not the only player in the game. The prefrontal cortex, with its cool, rational thinking, and the basal ganglia, with its ability to control our actions and thoughts, can work together to tame the amygdala's knee-jerk reactions.

So, the next time you find yourself in the grip of a sudden emotional outburst, take a deep breath and remember: you've got the power to outsmart your amygdala. After all, the best way to get rid of an angry amygdala is with a healthy dose of common sense and a good sense of humor.

CHAPTER 9

SENSORY RECEPTORS

Have you ever wondered how the human mind is able to accomplish such incredible feats - perceiving the world around us, understanding language, and deftly controlling our bodies? It's a process so seamless and natural that we often take it for granted. But delve a little deeper, and you'll uncover the remarkable mechanisms that make the mind work. Of course, its XCode all the way.

Let's start at the beginning. The origins of this remarkable mental machinery can be traced back to the earliest animals, even the humble Hydra. These simple, tubular creatures were controlled by a primitive neural network that could sense touch and trigger the appropriate muscular contractions. It was a rudimentary system, but one that foreshadowed the incredible complexity to come.

As evolution progressed, these neural networks grew more advanced, developing specialized receptors to detect a wider range of stimuli - light, sound, taste, and smell. Suddenly, these animals could perceive the world in vivid detail, and XCode enabled them to make sense of these sensory signals. A foul odor? XCode would instantly recognise it as a potential threat, triggering a reflexive recoil. A delicious morsel? XCode would coordinate the muscle movements to capture and consume it.

This pattern-recognition prowess only continued to expand over the eons, culminating in the remarkably sophisticated human mind. Our XCode powered brains can translate the most complex sensory inputs - the patterns of light on our retinas, the vibrations of sound waves, the subtle chemical signatures on our tongue - into a rich, multidimensional understanding of our environment.

But it doesn't stop there. XCode also underpins our capacity for emotion, memory, and higher cognition. The amygdala, for instance, uses this pattern-recognition system to rapidly detect signs of danger and trigger fear responses. The insula, meanwhile, taps into XCode's social intelligence to help us empathize with others and feel things like guilt, shame, and compassion.

Even our sense of self, our feeling of "I," emerges from the intricate interplay of XCode processes. The claustrum, a small but crucial structure, synthesizes sensory information to construct our conscious experience of the world and our place within it.

In essence, XCode is the unsung hero of the human mind - a silent, tireless worker that transforms the endless flood of sensory data into the rich, coherent reality we experience every day. It's a remarkable feat of pattern recognition, one that has been honed and refined over millions of years of evolution.

So the next time you effortlessly catch a ball, or instantly recognize a loved one's face, take a moment to appreciate the incredible power of XCode - the secret code that makes the human mind function with such elegance and efficiency. It's a testament to the astounding capabilities of our sensory receptors, and a humbling reminder of the depth and complexity of our own consciousness.

A THEORY OF HUMOR

Have you ever wondered why certain things strike us as hilarious, while others fall completely flat? Why does a slapstick mishap or a clever punchline have the power to make us erupt in side-splitting laughter, even against our will? The answer, my friends, lies in the remarkable inner workings of our own minds.

You see, the ability to recognize and appreciate humor is not just a quirky human behavior - it's a window into the very architecture of the brain itself. According to the "theory of humor" from Thomas, our capacity for laughter is rooted in the specialized, parallel processing capabilities of the two cerebral hemispheres.

Imagine, if you will, that your brain contains distinct functional regions, each with its own unique responsibilities. One of these key regions is responsible for interpreting emotions and making sense of the world around us. And this region is actually divided into two halves - the left and right hemispheres.

The left hemisphere is all about logical, rational thinking - the kind we rely on for our everyday routines and rituals. Meanwhile, the right hemisphere is specialized in handling unexpected or novel events, dealing with the emotional behaviors we exhibit in times of crisis or uncertainty.

This fundamental division between the two sides of the brain allows us to simultaneously evaluate the world from two radically different viewpoints. And it's this duality that lies at the heart of humor.

You see, humor arises when these two hemispheres reach conflicting interpretations of the same situation. The left brain might identify a "reason for tension" - a potential threat or source of discomfort. But the right brain, with its more logical pattern-recognition abilities, quickly realizes that the perceived threat is actually false or absurd.

It's this sudden shift in perspective, from tension to relaxation, that triggers the brain's laughter response. The amygdala, which detects emotional signals, springs into action, sending neural impulses that manifest as the uncontrollable giggles and chuckles we associate with humor.

Just imagine the scene: you're watching a classic Laurel and Hardy skit, where the bumbling duo get into one silly predicament after another. Your left brain acknowledges the potential for pain and peril, while your right brain can't help but recognize the utter absurdity of their antics. The result? You laugh.

Now, this whole process of humor might seem like just a quirky human trait. But the theory of humor actually suggests it may have evolutionary origins, dating back to our primal ancestors. You see, laughter and humor may have developed as a way for herd animals to identify and remember false alarms.

Imagine a young gazelle at play, blissfully unaware of a lurking predator. When one member of the herd detects the threat, the tension spreads through the group, triggering heightened vigilance. But when the danger is revealed to be a false alarm, the release of that tension is marked by shared laughter - a response that helps cement the memory and prevent unnecessary panic in the future.

So in a way, our capacity for humor is a testament to the extraordinary complexity and adaptability of the human brain. It's a trait that not only brings us joy and amusement, but also offers a glimpse into the neural underpinnings of our most fundamental cognitive processes.

The next time you find yourself in stitches over a well-timed punchline or a classic slapstick gag, take a moment to appreciate the remarkable interplay of brain regions at work. It's a reminder that the secrets to unlocking the mysteries of the mind may very well lie in the unexpected - and often hilarious - workings of our own gray matter. So go ahead, indulge in a good laugh. Your brain will thank you for it.

DETERMINISM VS FREE WILL

For centuries, philosophers and scientists have grappled with the age-old question - do we truly have free will, or are our thoughts and actions predetermined by forces beyond our control? It's a debate that goes to the heart of our understanding of human agency and moral responsibility. But what if you read here that the very notion of free will is nothing more than an illusion?

To understand this radical idea, let's dive into the concept of determinism. Fundamentally, determinism is the belief that everything that happens, including our choices and decisions, is the inevitable result of prior causes. As the ancient Stoic philosopher Chrysippus put it, "Everything that happens is followed by something else which depends on it by causal necessity." In other words, the universe is like a giant machine, with each event leading inexorably to the next in a never-ending chain of cause and effect.

Now, you might be thinking, "But wait, if everything is predetermined, how can I possibly have free will?" And that's a fair question. After all, the idea of determinism seems to directly undermine our cherished belief in autonomous decision-making. How can we be truly free if our choices are just the inevitable result of factors beyond our control?

Well, as it turns out, the reality may be even stranger than you think. You see, the more we learn about the inner workings of the human brain, the more it becomes clear that our conscious experience of decision-making is often just an illusion. Take the pioneering work of neuroscientist Benjamin Libet, who famously discovered that the neural precursors to our voluntary actions actually begin before we're even consciously aware of them.

Imagine you're sitting in a room, and you suddenly feel the urge to raise your hand. You think to yourself, "I'm going to raise my hand now." But Libet's experiments showed that the motor activity in your brain actually starts up to half a second before you become consciously aware of the decision. In other words, your brain is already setting the wheels in motion before you even realize what's happening.

So, if your conscious mind is just a passive observer, tagging along for the ride, where does that leave free will?

Well, according to some philosophers and scientists, it doesn't leave much room for it at all. As the renowned neuroscientist Sam Harris puts it, "You are not the author of your thoughts and actions in the way that a novelist is the author of a novel."

But wait, you might say, doesn't this contradict our everyday experience of making choices and being held accountable for our actions? Isn't that evidence of free will in action? Well, not necessarily. You see, the truth is that our brains are incredibly complex, with multiple systems and processes working together to guide our behavior.

Sure, the XCode - that incredible pattern-matching superpower we talked about before - is a key part of this. But there are also emotional drives, safety mechanisms, and other neural subsystems that are constantly shaping our decisions, often without our conscious awareness. It's like your brain is a bustling committee, with various factions vying for control, and your conscious self is just the chairperson, tasked with making sense of it all.

So, what are we to make of all this? Does the evidence for determinism mean that we're all just biochemical puppets, doomed to act out a script we had no hand in writing? Well, not necessarily. Even if our choices aren't the result of some mythical "free will," that doesn't mean we're completely powerless. After all, the ability to examine our own thought processes, to reflect on our actions, and to strive to become better versions of ourselves - that's a pretty remarkable feat in its own right.

And who knows, maybe there's a middle ground to be found between the rigid determinism of the universe and the free-wheeling notion of absolute free will. Perhaps, as the philosopher Rudolf Steiner suggested, true freedom lies in aligning our choices with our moral imagination and ethical ideals. Or maybe, as the Buddhists have long taught, the path to liberation is through the cultivation of self-awareness and the quieting of our turbulent emotions.

It's true that our brain uses what Thomas calls the "WASP" criteria - Worthwhile, Appropriate, Safe, and Practical considerations - to make decisions, and that our emotions can often overwhelm our best intentions. But we have the power to draw the attention of the mind and direct it towards greater wisdom.

By educating our minds and deliberately focusing our attention on the prudence of good choices, we can help shape the automatic mechanisms of XCode that the limbic system uses to guide our thoughts and behaviors. Instead of being at the mercy of our emotional impulses, we can harness the incredible power of this hidden decision-making hub to lead us along wise paths. The real challenge, Thomas suggests, lies in embracing the mystery of our minds, finding agency within the apparent constraints of our circumstances, and using the full capacities of our consciousness to thoughtfully shape the future, one decision at a time.

DEFINE COMMON SENSE

When it comes to the concept of "common sense," it's amazing how much confusion and misunderstanding there is. People bandy the term around all the time, as if it's this universally understood idea. But the truth is, science has struggled to clearly define what common sense really is. Even philosophers tend to avoid the phrase, finding it too vague and imprecise.

But here's the thing - just because common sense is tough to pin down, doesn't mean it's not an incredibly important and powerful aspect of the human mind. In fact, Thomas argues that common sense is one of the key drivers behind our ability to navigate the world and make sound decisions. And the good news is, we can all tap into this inner wellspring of wisdom - we just need to understand how it works.

You see, at the core of common sense is the prefrontal region of the brain - the part that's responsible for that cool, calm, and collected way of looking at things. Now, this isn't the same as the more emotional, reactive parts of the brain, like the limbic system. No, the prefrontal regions are all about integration, analysis, and unemotional evaluation.

It's like your brain has these two control centers - one that's driven by gut feelings, fears, and other primal impulses, and another that's all about rational, big-picture thinking. And the secret to tapping into true common sense is learning how to quiet down that emotional side and let the prefrontal regions take the wheel.

Now, you might be thinking, "But wait, if common sense is just the output of one part of the brain, how can it be 'common' to everyone?" And that's a fair point. After all, the dictionary definition of common sense suggests that it's this universally shared, basic understanding that we all just kind of "get."

But the reality is, common sense is actually quite personal and individualized. What might seem like obvious, prudent judgment to one person could come across as downright stupidity to another. It all comes down to the unique information and life experiences that each of us has access to.

Just imagine two people looking at the same situation - say, a broken appliance that needs fixing. One person might immediately see the solution, drawing on their wealth of technical knowledge and past repair experiences. The other, well, they might just be scratching their head, feeling utterly flummoxed. Same situation, vastly different common sense perspectives.

And that's the key thing to understand - common sense isn't about some universal set of rules or logical propositions. No, it's about the calm, unemotional way that your prefrontal regions process and integrate all the sensory information flooding into your brain. It's about taking a step back, quieting the noise of your emotional impulses, and trying to see the situation for what it truly is.

Now, you might be wondering, "If common sense is so personal and individualized, how can it be a reliable guide for decision-making?" And that's a fair question. After all, if everyone's common sense is different, how can we trust it to lead us in the right direction?

Well, the answer lies in the power of self-awareness and the cultivation of emotional control. You see, the more we're able to quiet down the reactive, knee-jerk parts of our brain, the more we can tap into the clear-headed, big-picture perspective of our prefrontal regions. And the more we do that, the more our common sense starts to align with true wisdom, tact, and good judgment.

It's a bit like training a wild horse - at first, it's all about managing the animal's primal instincts and impulses. But over time, as calm controls build trust and understanding, that horse becomes a powerful, reliable partner, guided by a calm, collected way of being in the world. And the same goes for our own minds - the more we cultivate self-awareness and emotional control, the more our common sense can shine through as a beacon of clarity and sound decision-making.

The foundation of common sense lies in its roots in the prefrontal regions. The limbic system, which includes the amygdala and insula, is directly connected and serves as the driving force behind our intuitive, emotionally-charged decisions. These areas contain the memories and experiences that trigger our emotional responses, shaping our gut instincts and emotional judgments.

In contrast, the prefrontal regions of the brain have fewer direct links to the limbic system, allowing them to process emotional signals without being fully immersed in the physical sensations. This separation enables the prefrontal cortex to make more unemotional, rational assessments, tempering the impulsive tendencies of the limbic system. XCode triggers emotions when the limbic system is in charge and common sense when the prefrontal regions take control..

And who knows, maybe as we continue to explore and understand the incredible complexity of the human brain, we'll unlock even greater secrets about stilling the mind to place common sense in charge. Because at the end of the day, that's what true intelligence is all about - not just the ability to crunch numbers or win at trivia, but the wisdom to navigate the challenges of life with clarity, compassion, and a healthy dose of that elusive, yet oh-so-powerful common sense.

CHAPTER 13

HUMAN MEMORY RESEARCH MISTAKE

You know, when it comes to the human brain, we tend to get pretty dazzled by all the flashy stuff - the lightning-fast pattern recognition of XCode, the neuronal intelligence that allows us to navigate the social world, and of course, lets us solve complex problems and come up with brilliant ideas.

But you know what often gets overlooked in all the hype? The mind-boggling, awe-inspiring capacity of human memory. I mean, think about it - we're talking about a system that can store and recall trillions upon trillions of sensory experiences, from the smell of grandma's famous apple pie to the intricate muscle movements required to play a

Beethoven sonata. It's like our brains are these colossal libraries, filled to the brim with volumes upon volumes of meticulously organized information.

And yet, for all the incredible feats of memory we're capable of, the scientific community has kind of dropped the ball when it comes to really understanding how it all works. I mean, sure, we know about things like long-term potentiation (LTP) and the role of the hippocampus in storing contextual memories. But when you really start to dive into the sheer scale and precision of human memory, it becomes clear that there's a whole lot more going on beneath the surface.

Take, for example, the mind-blowing fact that the average person can actually differentiate between up to 1 trillion distinct smells. That's a number so staggeringly large, it's hard to even wrap your head around it. And it's not just about smells - our brains are capable of storing and recalling millions upon millions of images, as well as the intricate sequences of muscle movements required for everything from running to speaking.

So, what's the deal? Why has science been so quick to dismiss the true genius of human memory as just a bunch of simple "Dial 100" responses, or the result of a few measly branches growing on our neurons? I mean, come on, do they really think the combined wisdom of millions of years of evolution can be boiled down to something that simplistic?

The truth is, I think the problem lies in the way scientists have traditionally approached the study of memory. They've been so focused on the nitty-gritty details - the specific molecules, the neural pathways, the behavioral experiments - that they've lost sight of the big picture. They're like a bunch of archaeologists, painstakingly excavating individual shards of pottery, without ever stepping back to admire the grand, sprawling civilization that once thrived there.

But what if we took a different approach? What if, instead of getting bogged down in the mathematical minutiae, we started to view the human brain as the incredible pattern-recognition machine that it is? Because make no mistake, that's what's really going on here - our neurons aren't just passive computational units, they're dynamic, adaptable systems that are constantly scanning, learning, and creating intricate, combinatorial webs of memories.

Imagine your brain as this vast, interconnected library, filled with trillions of volumes, each one a unique sensory experience or learned skill. And every time a new piece of information comes in, your neurons are furiously flipping through those pages, searching for matches, making connections, and forging new pathways. It's like a symphony of pattern recognition, playing out at a scale that would make even the most powerful supercomputer green with envy.

And you know what's really wild? This incredible memory capacity isn't just about being able to recall the details of last week's dinner or that catchy pop song you heard on the radio. No, it's also the foundation for all of our other mental abilities - our capacity for learning, our social and emotional intelligence, even our capacity for creativity and problem-solving. Because when you think about it, every time you have a sudden flash of insight or a burst of inspiration, it's your memory system working its magic, drawing on that vast trove of accumulated knowledge and experience.

So, the next time you find yourself marveling at someone's "genius," or feeling a bit down about your own cognitive prowess, remember - the true mark of intelligence isn't just about academic achievements or logical reasoning. It's about the sheer, awe-inspiring capacity of the human mind to store, process, and retrieve information on a scale that's almost impossible to fathom. And that, my friends, is something we should all be incredibly proud of.

Who knows, maybe one day we'll unlock the secrets of XCode and be able to harness its power in ways we can scarcely imagine. But for now, let's just take a moment to appreciate XCode - the quiet, unsung brilliance of our own mental libraries - the trillions of sensory experiences, the millions of learned skills, the endless web of patterns and connections that make us who we are. Because when you really think about it, that's the true essence of intelligence - not just the ability to solve problems, but the capacity to remember, to learn, and to grow, one moment at a time.

CHAPTER 14

HUMAN MEMORY CAPACITY

Have you ever wondered how your brain is able to recognize a face in the blink of an eye? Or how a skilled perfumer can distinguish between over a trillion unique scents? The conventional view of intelligence as logical reasoning and problem-solving just doesn't seem to capture the true marvel of the human mind.

Let me take you on a journey through the hidden depths of our mental capacities, where pattern recognition and evolutionary biology intertwine to reveal a radically different understanding of intelligence.

Imagine for a moment the brain of a mouse - a tiny, unassuming creature that can detect and distinguish between countless odors with astounding precision. It turns out that the key to this remarkable olfactory ability lies in the combinatorial coding of its olfactory neurons.

Each receptor cell in the mouse's nose is attuned to recognize a specific set of odor molecules. When these molecules bind to the receptors, they trigger unique combinations of neuron firings that the brain can then interpret as distinct smells.

In a groundbreaking experiment, researchers used calcium imaging to observe these patterns of neuronal activation. They found that a single receptor cell could identify multiple odors, while a single odor was recognized by the combined firing of several receptor cells. This "alphabet" of olfactory receptors allowed the mouse's brain to build an incredibly detailed and vast "vocabulary" of scents - an estimated one trillion unique smells that the humble mouse can readily distinguish.

Now, let's zoom out and consider the implications of this discovery. If a tiny mouse brain can store and retrieve such an astronomical amount of sensory information, just imagine the capacity of the human mind. Indeed, studies have shown that ordinary people can instantly recognize billions of visual pixels, identifying any of 10,000 images shown to them at 1 second intervals with 99.5% accuracy. The secret lies in the power of combinatorial coding - the brain's ability to effortlessly weave together intricate patterns of neuronal activity to represent and remember an almost infinite number of sensory experiences.

So the next time you effortlessly recall a face, savor a fine wine, or navigate a familiar landscape, remember that your mind is tapping into vast combinatorially coded neuronal memories stored in the 20 micrometer spaces of 86 billion neurons. A vast repertoire of evolutionary memories, weaving together intricate patterns of neuronal activity to create the rich tapestry of your lived experience. Intelligence, it seems, is not what we thought it was - it's something far more extraordinary and mysterious, a quantum symphony that continues to captivate and inspire us.

CHAPTER 15

THE INSULAR CORTEX

Have you ever had one of those moments where you just instinctively knew the right thing to do, even if you couldn't fully explain why? Or found yourself experiencing a strong emotional reaction - maybe a twinge of disgust or a swell of empathy - that seemed to arise from deep within? If so, you were likely experiencing the remarkable power of the insular cortex, a little-known region of the brain that plays a surprisingly crucial role in our daily lives.

The insular cortex is sometimes described as the "underdog" of the brain - overshadowed by the glitz and glamor of other more famous areas like the prefrontal cortex and the amygdala. But as we'll soon see, this unassuming part of our gray matter is absolutely essential for things like self-awareness, social intelligence, and moral decision-making. In fact, you could say the insular cortex is the secret superhero of the human mind.

Let's start with how the insular cortex helps us develop a sense of self. Imagine for a moment that you're reaching out to touch a hot stovetop. Even before your finger makes contact, your brain is already sending out warning signals - a tingle of anticipated pain. That's thanks to the insular cortex, which acts as a sort of control center, constantly monitoring the sensations and movements of our physical bodies.

The insular cortex allows us to perceive our bodies as a unified "self" - not just a jumble of disconnected parts and sensations. It's what gives us that gut-level awareness of our own existence. And research has shown that damage to the insular cortex can profoundly disrupt this sense of self, leading to a feeling of alienation from one's own body. Lesions in the organ had caused a patient to believe that his own hand did not belong to him!

But the insular cortex does more than just make us self-aware - it also allows us to empathize with others. You know that pang of sympathy you feel when you see someone else in pain? That's the insular cortex at work, firing up the same neural pathways that would be activated if you were experiencing that pain yourself. It's like a neural mirror, allowing us to truly "feel" what others are going through.

This empathetic capacity is crucial for navigating the complex social world. After all, how can we hope to cooperate and collaborate with our fellow humans if we can't even begin to understand what they're feeling? The insular cortex is what gives us that innate social glue, helping to bind us together as a species.

And the insular cortex doesn't stop there. It also plays a key role in our moral decision-making, helping us to distinguish right from wrong. Remember that visceral feeling of disgust you get when you witness something truly reprehensible? That's the insular cortex at work again, triggering a physical rejection response to moral transgressions.

In a way, the insular cortex is like a highly sophisticated bouncer, constantly scanning the social landscape and giving us those gut-level cues about what's acceptable and what's not. It's what allows us to develop a strong moral compass and internal sense of right and wrong.

But what exactly is the insular cortex "listening" to, in order to generate all these intuitive responses? The answer lies in the vast network of nerve cells that constantly transmit information about the state of our bodies to this remarkable brain region.

Specialized neurons detect everything from temperature and touch to pain, itch, and changes in oxygen levels, sending a ceaseless stream of sensory data to the insula. It's like a symphony of bodily signals, all feeding into the insular cortex's central processing unit.

And the insula doesn't just passively receive this information - it actively interprets and responds to it. For example, the insula can recognize specific patterns of nerve cell activity that indicate the presence of rotten or contaminated food, triggering a disgust response to protect us from harm.

Or it can detect signals of pleasure or distress in others, allowing us to empathize with their experiences. In a sense, the nerve cells reporting to the insula are the insular cortex's eyes and ears, giving it a rich, multidimensional understanding of both our own bodies and the world around us. This continuous flow of sensory data is what empowers the insula to fulfill its vital functions in self-awareness, social cognition, and moral reasoning.

So the next time you find yourself making a snap judgment or experiencing a sudden emotional reaction, take a moment to appreciate the hidden power of the insular cortex. This unsung hero of the brain is constantly working behind the scenes, using a vast repertoire of evolutionary memories and pattern-recognition skills to guide us through the complex social world.

It just goes to show that true intelligence isn't always what it seems on the surface. Sometimes, the most important cognitive functions are happening in the quieter, more unassuming corners of the brain. The insular cortex may be small, but its impact is anything but.

CHAPTER 16

MIRROR NEURONS

Have you ever felt a pang of sadness when seeing a friend go through a difficult time? Or winced in sympathetic pain when watching someone get hurt? These powerful emotional responses happen thanks to an incredible neural network in our brains called the mirror system. This mirror network is a perfect illustration of the concept of XCode.

Let me paint you a picture. Imagine you're at a party, chatting with a group of friends. As you're talking, you notice one of your friends make a pained expression. Without even thinking about it, you feel a twinge of discomfort in your own body. It's as if you can almost sense their pain as your own. This remarkable phenomenon is all thanks to a fascinating class of brain cells called mirror neurons.

These special neurons, first discovered in the 1990s, don't just light up when we perform an action ourselves - they also activate when we observe someone else doing the same thing. It's as if our brain has a neural "mirroring" system that allows us to instantly experience and understand the intentions, emotions, and sensations of those around us, almost as if we're walking a mile in their shoes. This is a prime example of the XCode system in action - our brains rapidly associating the visual cues we see with our own stored sensory-motor memories to create an embodied, experiential understanding.

The implications of this mirror network are profound. It suggests that our intelligence and social understanding goes far beyond just thinking and reasoning. In fact, the bulk of our knowledge about the world and other people comes not from conscious thought, but from this deep, intuitive, subconscious process of pattern recognition and embodied simulation - hallmarks of the XCode framework.

Just consider how much we glean from simple things like a friend's facial expression or body language. Studies show that less than 10% of our social understanding comes from actual words - the rest comes from this implicit mirroring process. Our mirror neurons allow us to rapidly decode the unspoken emotions and intentions of others, giving us a rich, experiential understanding that goes beyond mere logical deduction.

This concept flies in the face of the traditional view of intelligence as purely analytical and rational. Instead, it paints a picture of the human mind as an incredible pattern-matching machine, drawing on vast evolutionary libraries of embodied knowledge to instantly make sense of the social world around us. It's like we have a hidden superpower - the ability to intuitively grasp the experiences of others, almost as if we can single-handedly step into their shoes.

And the applications of this mirror network go far beyond just social understanding. Studies have shown that these neurons are involved in everything from learning new physical skills to empathizing with the pain of others. A musician, for example, may unconsciously "mirror" the movements of a virtuoso they're watching, allowing them to more easily learn the technique. And people who report higher levels of empathy tend to have stronger activations in their mirror systems when observing emotional states.

So the next time you find yourself inexplicably yawning after seeing someone else do it, or cringing in sympathy at the sight of someone stubbing their toe, remember - it's not just your imagination. It's your mirror neurons at work, giving you a seamless, embodied understanding of the world and the people around you. Perhaps intelligence isn't what we thought it was after all - it's a deep, intuitive, pattern-matching superpower that we all possess, rooted in the XCode framework that underlies so much of our cognitive abilities. It's a hidden power that allows us to transcend the limits of logic and truly connect with the experiences of others.

CHAPTER 17

THE SOCIAL COMPARISON THEORY

Have you ever found yourself inexplicably drawn to compare your achievements, possessions, or social status to those around you? Perhaps you felt a pang of envy when a neighbor got a shiny new car, or a twinge of frustration when a coworker received a promotion you had your eye on. These subtle emotional responses are the product of a powerful, yet hidden mental mechanism known as social comparison.

Just as XCode works behind the scenes to shape our cognitive abilities, the social comparison process operates as an ever-present, subconscious driver of our behavior. It's a relentless force that has been honed by evolution to help us navigate the complex social hierarchies of our communities.

Imagine a herd of grazing animals, huddled together for safety on the open plains. As they move and act in sync, their individual behaviors are not governed by a centralized plan, but by an intricate web of social cues and comparisons. The animals instinctively monitor each other, seeking to align their actions with the "leaders" of the group. This allows the herd to function as a cohesive unit, maximizing their chances of survival.

In much the same way, our own nervous systems are constantly scanning the people around us, making subtle comparisons that shape our emotions and actions. Step into an elevator, and you'll likely feel your muscles stiffen, keeping a respectful distance from your fellow passengers. Wander into a museum, and your voice will automatically lower to match the formal atmosphere. This social sensitivity is not a conscious choice, but an ingrained response driven by the social comparison process.

The concept of social comparison was first proposed by social psychologist Leon Festinger in 1954. Festinger theorized that individuals have an innate drive to evaluate their own opinions and abilities by comparing themselves to others. This drive, he argued, is a fundamental part of the human psyche, helping us to make sense of our place within the social hierarchy.

At its core, this drive to evaluate ourselves against others is rooted in the fundamental human need to belong and fit into our social groups. By constantly benchmarking our wealth, status, and abilities against our perceived "equals," we are able to assess our standing within the hierarchy and adjust our behavior accordingly. The fear of being ostracized or rejected by the group was a matter of life and death for our ancestors, and this primal survival instinct remains deeply wired into our psyche.

However, this ceaseless process of social comparison can also be a double-edged sword. While it may motivate us to improve our performance and strive for greater achievements, it can also trigger a host of negative emotions, from envy and anger to shame and despair. When we see someone who appears to be outperforming us, our subconscious mind springs into action, generating bodily responses that prepare us for a "fight or flight" scenario. Our heart rates increase, our muscles tense, and a flood of adrenaline courses through our veins - all before we're even consciously aware of what's happening.

These emotional reactions are not the result of logic or rational thinking, but rather the product of a deeply ingrained pattern recognition process. Our minds are constantly scanning the behavior of those around us, comparing our own traits and abilities to those of our peers. And when we perceive a discrepancy, our bodies respond with a suite of primal emotional responses, designed to spur us into action.

The problem is, in the modern world, these emotional triggers are often misaligned with our actual circumstances. A person may feel ashamed about their financial situation, even though they have access to resources and opportunities that previous generations could only dream of. Or they may experience crippling envy towards a neighbor's material possessions, without fully appreciating the hard work and sacrifices that went into acquiring them.

Fortunately, there is a way to mitigate the negative impacts of social comparison. By developing a deeper understanding of this subconscious process, and cultivating a greater sense of self-awareness, we can learn to temper our emotional reactions and redirect our focus towards more constructive goals.

One key strategy is to consciously expose ourselves to realistic, achievable comparisons. When we set our sights on benchmarks that are within reach, we are more likely to experience the positive motivational effects of social comparison, rather than being mired in feelings of despair or resentment. Additionally, by practicing mindfulness and paying close attention to the physical sensations and emotional responses triggered by social comparisons, we can learn to observe them with detachment, rather than becoming overwhelmed by them.

Ultimately, the social comparison process is a testament to the incredible complexity and adaptability of the human mind. It is a mechanism that has evolved to help us navigate the social world, but one that can also lead us astray if left unchecked. By understanding its inner workings and learning to harness its power, we can unlock new realms of personal growth and fulfillment, and forge a more harmonious relationship with the world around us.

CHAPTER 18

LONG TERM POTENTIATION

It was 1973, and Terje Lømo, a young Norwegian neuroscientist, was busy tinkering away in his lab at the University of Oslo. Lømo was fascinated by the inner workings of the brain and how it processed information, storing it away for future recall. At the time, the prevailing theory was that memories were stored through changes in the strength of connections between neurons - a process known as synaptic plasticity.

Lømo had been experimenting with electrically stimulating the nerve pathways in the brains of rabbits, trying to understand how these connections strengthened and weakened over time. One day, as he was delivering a high-frequency burst of electrical pulses to a particular neural pathway, something remarkable happened.

Instead of the typical short-lived increase in the strength of the connection, Lømo observed that the effect persisted for hours, even days! It was as if the neurons had "remembered" the initial stimulation, becoming more responsive to subsequent signals. Lømo couldn't believe his eyes - he had stumbled upon a phenomenon that would go on to revolutionize our understanding of how the brain stores and retrieves memories.

Lømo likened this discovery to a "speed dial" for the brain's memory system. Imagine your old rotary-dial phone, where you had to painstakingly spin the dial to reach a specific number. Long-term potentiation, or LTP as it would come to be known, was like a direct line that allowed the brain to quickly and efficiently access important information.

Just as a speed dial bypasses the laborious process of dialing a number, LTP streamlined the brain's ability to recall critical memories. It was as if the neurons had been rewired to create a more efficient pathway, making it easier for the brain to access and retrieve those crucial pieces of information.

Lømo's discovery was the first concrete evidence that the brain could actively modify the strength of its connections in response to specific experiences. This process, known as synaptic plasticity, was a far cry from the traditional view of the brain as a static, unchanging organ. Instead, it revealed the brain's remarkable ability to adapt and evolve, constantly rewiring itself to better suit the needs of the individual.

As news of Lømo's findings spread, the scientific community was abuzz with excitement. Here was a mechanism that could potentially explain how the brain stores and recalls memories, a fundamental question that had puzzled researchers for decades. Lømo's accidental discovery had opened up a whole new frontier in the study of the mind, one that would lead to a deeper understanding of the brain's incredible capacity for learning and adaptation.

Of course, the story of LTP didn't end there. In the years that followed, researchers around the world would build upon Lømo's work, uncovering the intricate molecular mechanisms that underlie this phenomenon. They would discover that LTP wasn't just a quirky side effect, but a critical component of the brain's memory-making machinery.

As we delve deeper into the fascinating world of the XCode, Lømo's serendipitous finding will serve as a reminder that the most groundbreaking discoveries often happen when we least expect them. By keeping an open mind and a curious spirit, we just might stumble upon the key that unlocks the secrets of the mind.

BEHAVIOR PATTERN RECOGNITION

Imagine you're a security agent at a busy airport, tasked with identifying potential threats before they can cause harm. Your eyes scan the crowds, searching for any suspicious behaviors - a person lingering nervously near the checkpoints, a bead of sweat trickling down a tense brow, a subtle hand signal exchanged between two individuals. It's a complex puzzle, piecing together these subtle cues into a coherent picture of what's really going on.

This kind of "behavior pattern recognition" isn't just the purview of security experts - it's a fundamental function of the human mind, one that allows us to make sense of the endless flow of information we encounter every day. From the moment we wake up to the time we go to sleep, our brains are constantly processing a dizzying array of sights, sounds, and sensations, extracting meaningful patterns from the chaos.

How exactly does this remarkable feat of pattern recognition work? To understand it, let's take a step back and consider a simpler example - the way our minds recognize different smells and tastes. Scientists have discovered that the olfactory and gustatory systems in our brains employ a clever "combinatorial coding" strategy, where individual receptor neurons fire in unique combinations to identify specific odorants or molecules.

It's a bit like a security system that uses a series of checkpoints, each with its own set of criteria, to determine if a potential threat is present. Just as airport scanners look for a confluence of suspicious behaviors, our sensory receptors look for the right combination of chemical signals to identify a particular scent or flavor. And the more receptors involved, the more nuanced and precise the recognition becomes.

But the human mind doesn't stop at simply identifying individual stimuli - it also has the remarkable ability to recognize complex sequences and patterns over time. Imagine a dog sniffing out a trail, using the subtle differences in odor intensity to determine the direction a person has walked. Or picture yourself navigating through a busy city, effortlessly tracking the movements of cars, pedestrians, and traffic signals - a dizzying array of dynamic information that your brain organizes into a coherent mental map.

This dynamic recognition process is akin to watching a movie, where each frame is a unique snapshot, but the full sequence tells a story. Just as a film's subtitles can label and identify the action unfolding on the screen, our brains attach labels and meanings to the sensory information we encounter, creating a rich tapestry of understanding.

And it's not just simple actions like "sitting" or "running" that our minds can recognize - we're capable of comprehending far more complex behavioral patterns, from the nuances of human language to the intricate strategies of war. Each sentence, each plan, each theory is a unique combination of words, ideas, and relationships, woven together into a meaningful whole.

It's a mind-boggling feat of neural engineering, one that draws upon vast libraries of memories and associations stored deep within our brains. Just as a computer system would require terabytes of data to simulate the breadth and depth of human knowledge, our own minds rely on an almost incomprehensible amount of information to make sense of the world around us.

But the real power of behavior pattern recognition lies not just in its sheer scale, but in its adaptability and flexibility. Our brains are constantly learning, constantly updating their internal models to account for new experiences and insights. A single frame of a movie may be meaningless on its own, but when viewed in the context of the entire film, it takes on new depth and significance.

So, the next time you find yourself effortlessly navigating a crowded room, or intuitively understanding the subtle subtext of a conversation, take a moment to appreciate the incredible feat of pattern recognition happening beneath the surface. It's a testament to the remarkable capabilities of the human mind - a mind that, in many ways, puts even the most advanced artificial intelligence systems to shame.

CHAPTER 20

THE ORIENTING RESPONSE

Have you ever been zoning out, lost in your own thoughts, when suddenly a loud noise or bright flash jolts you back to attention? That's your brain's orienting response at work - an evolutionary mechanism that compels us to focus on new and important information, even before we fully process what it is.

The orienting response is like a built-in "opportunity detector" that hones in on changes in our environment. It's a crucial survival mechanism, evolved to ensure we don't miss out on critical new information that could impact our wellbeing or success. And understanding how this response functions offers a fascinating glimpse into the true nature of human intelligence.

You see, the conventional view of intelligence is far too narrow. It's typically defined by static measures like IQ tests - a snapshot in time that fails to capture the dynamic, adaptable nature of the human mind. But the orienting response reveals something much more profound about how our brains actually work.

Imagine you're out on a nature hike, peacefully taking in the sights and sounds around you. Suddenly, a twig snaps in the distance. Immediately, your gaze is drawn to the source of the noise, your senses heightened, your mind racing to assess the potential threat or opportunity. This is your orienting response in action.

Within seconds, your brain has carried out a complex series of activities. Skin conductance, brain waves, and heart rate all shift, priming your body for action. Deeper in the brain, the hippocampus, anterior cingulate, and prefrontal cortex spring into motion, rapidly sifting through memories and evaluating the significance of the new stimulus.

But the orienting response isn't just about survival. It's also a gateway to personal growth and achievement. You see, this response doesn't just alert us to danger - it also draws our attention to novel situations that could be beneficial, like a promising job opportunity or a chance to learn a new skill.

Imagine you're browsing the internet and stumble upon an article about a fascinating new field you've never heard of before. Your eyes might linger on the page, your mind captivated by the possibilities. That's your orienting response at work, compelling you to explore this novel information that could open up new horizons.

The truly remarkable thing is that the orienting response is intricately linked to our emotions and memories. The intensity of our emotional reaction to a new stimulus directly influences how strongly the orienting response is triggered. And those gaze patterns we exhibit when we're captivated by something? They get recorded in the brain, forming the basis of our memories and guiding our future behavior.

It's as if our brains are wired to seek out the things that are most relevant and valuable to us as individuals. The orienting response is constantly scanning our environment, hunting for opportunities that align with our unique talents, interests, and life purpose. It's a dynamic, ever-evolving process that defies simplistic notions of intelligence.

So the next time you find yourself inexplicably drawn to a new idea or experience, don't dismiss it as a mere distraction. Embrace it as a sign that your brain's opportunity detector has been activated, guiding you towards personal growth and fulfillment. Because true intelligence isn't about static test scores - it's about the agility and adaptability to seize the moments that shape our lives.

TALLER THAN A TREE

With a chuckle, I'll leave you with a bit of wit to ponder: What's the difference between a laser and a mentally-focused individual? A laser beams, but a person orients.

CHAPTER 21

THE SOMATIC MARKER HYPOTHESIS

Have you ever wondered why some decisions feel like a no-brainer, while others leave you agonizing for hours? Or why certain situations just seem to trigger a visceral reaction in your gut, even if you can't quite explain why? The answer, my friends, lies in a fascinating neurological phenomenon known as the somatic marker hypothesis.

Let's dive in with a classic example. Imagine you're playing a high-stakes gambling game, choosing cards from different decks. Some decks offer big rewards, but also huge penalties. Other decks have smaller payouts, but the losses are more manageable. Over time, most people start to instinctively gravitate towards the safer, lower-risk decks -

but they can't always explain why. Their logical mind is telling them to keep chasing the bigger rewards, but their intuition is urging them in the opposite direction.

This is where the somatic marker hypothesis comes into play. According to this theory, proposed by renowned neuroscientist Antonio Damasio, our brains are constantly generating "somatic markers" - subtle bodily signals that act as emotional flags, guiding our decision-making.

Imagine your brain as a vast, interconnected command center, with different regions responsible for various functions. The ventromedial prefrontal cortex, or VMPFC, acts as a sort of emotional archivist, storing the bodily sensations associated with your past experiences. So when you're facing a high-risk decision in the gambling game, your VMPFC draws on those stored "somatic markers" - a queasy stomach, a racing heartbeat, a sense of dread - to steer you away from the dangerous decks, even if you can't consciously articulate why.

Patients with damage to the VMPFC, on the other hand, lack access to those crucial somatic markers. In the gambling experiment, they continued making risky choices, seemingly oblivious to the mounting losses. Their logical faculties were intact, but without the intuitive, gut-level guidance of the somatic markers, they struggled to make advantageous decisions.

It's a fascinating example of how our emotions and bodily sensations are inextricably linked to our decision-making process. The somatic marker hypothesis suggests that these physical signals - a quickening pulse, a clenched stomach, a surge of excitement - aren't just reactions to our choices, but active players in shaping them.

Imagine your brain as a high-powered supercomputer, processing trillions of bits of information in the blink of an eye. The somatic markers act as a sort of real-time feedback loop, constantly updating the system with emotional context and directing the flow of data. It's the difference between coldly weighing the pros and cons, and intuitively knowing what just "feels right."

Of course, that's not to say we should completely abandon logic and reason. The optimal approach is often a harmonious partnership between the rational and the intuitive. But by understanding the role of somatic markers, we can learn to harness the incredible power of our gut feelings, and tap into the hidden depths of human intelligence.

So the next time you're facing a tough decision, pay attention to those physical sensations. Is your heart racing? Is your stomach in knots? Those could be your somatic markers trying to guide you, drawing on a lifetime of emotional experiences to point you towards the wisest course of action. It may not be the answer your conscious mind expected, but trust that your intuition knows something your logic has yet to uncover.

The human brain is a magnificent, mysterious organ, capable of feats of brilliance that often defy explanation. The somatic marker hypothesis is just one glimpse into the incredible complexity and adaptability of this remarkable machine. So the next time you have a gut feeling, don't dismiss it - it might just be the key to unlocking your full potential.

CHAPTER 22

THE SAVANT BRAIN

Have you ever met someone who could do incredible feats of memory, calculation, or creativity - and then struggled with the most basic everyday tasks? These individuals, known as savants, provide a fascinating window into the hidden potential of the human brain.

Take the case of Raymond Babbitt, the character portrayed by Dustin Hoffman in the classic film Rain Man. Raymond could instantly recall the license plate numbers of every car he'd seen, recite the contents of a phone book from memory, and count the exact number of toothpicks that spilled on the floor. Yet, he had profound difficulties with social interaction and daily living skills.

How is this possible? The key lies in the remarkable way the savant brain processes and stores information. You see, while most of us rely on xCode to quickly access and apply general knowledge, savants have an unbalanced version of this system - one that has been taken over by a specific domain, like math or music.

Imagine your brain as a vast library, filled with countless books on every subject imaginable. In a typical brain, the XCode allows you to rapidly retrieve the relevant information you need, whether it's the capital of France or how to tie your shoelaces. But in a savant, one section of the library has become so dominant that it dwarfs all the others.

Take the case of the "calculating twins," as described by neurologist Oliver Sacks. These individuals could effortlessly rattle off prime numbers, as if the concepts were simply appearing in their minds. That's because their brains had dedicated an enormous amount of neural real estate to the study of mathematics, at the expense of other cognitive functions.

The key to this specialized brilliance lies in the way savant brains store and recall information. Rather than relying on the typical contextual hooks we use to remember things, savants build memories of limited subjects in regions wee use for other purposes. They build incredibly detailed, interconnected patterns of neural activity that allow them to instantly recognize and recall vast amounts of data in a narrow field.

Imagine you're trying to remember a phone number. Most of us would associate the digits with a person's name, their address, or some other contextual cue. But a savant might simply have a neural pattern that corresponds to that specific phone number, allowing them to recall it with lightning speed and perfect accuracy.

This phenomenon is not limited to savants. In fact, we all have the capacity to form these kinds of hyper-specific memories, if we focus our attention intensely enough on a subject. Think about how a doctor can spot a rare medical condition with a single glance, or how a musician can instantly recall the notes of a complex piece of music.

The savant brain, then, is not so much a distinct type of intelligence as it is an extreme example of the human brain's incredible capacity for pattern recognition and recall. By dedicating immense neural resources to a narrow domain, these individuals are able to unlock capabilities that most of us can only dream of.

But there's a trade-off. While savants excel in their areas of expertise, they often struggle with more general cognitive functions, like social skills and everyday tasks. Their hyper-focused brains have essentially sacrificed breadth for depth, leaving them vulnerable in areas outside their specialized knowledge.

So, the next time you meet someone with an uncanny talent, remember that they're not displaying a fundamentally different kind of intelligence - they're simply manifestations of the brain's incredible plasticity and power. With the right focus and dedication, we all have the potential to unlock our own extraordinary mental abilities.

And who knows? Maybe someday, we'll all be able to recite the phone book from memory. Though, personally, I'd be happier if I could just remember where I left my car keys.

THE MEANING OF CONSCIOUSNESS

Imagine you're walking through a park on a spring day. As you stroll, you take in the vibrant green of the leaves, the gentle breeze caressing your skin, the chirping of the birds, the sweet scent of blooming flowers. Your brain isn't processing each of those sensory inputs in isolation - it's weaving them together into a cohesive, integrated perception of your environment.

One of the key insights about consciousness comes from the work of researcher Nouchine Hadjikhani and her team. Using PET scans, they were able to identify a crucial role for a brain region called the claustrum in the way we consciously perceive the world around us.

The claustrum is a thin, sheet-like structure that sits deep within the brain, serving as a hub that connects to various sensory, motor, and emotional processing areas. Hadjikhani's research showed that the claustrum is particularly important for what scientists call "cross-modal matching" - the ability to integrate information from multiple senses simultaneously.

According to Hadjikhani's findings, the claustrum plays a crucial role in this cross-modal integration. By serving as a hub that connects all these different sensory regions, the claustrum is able to match up the patterns of neural activity, allowing you to experience the world as a unified, multi-dimensional whole.

Without the claustrum, Hadjikhani's research suggests, a person may still be able to respond to simple, familiar stimuli. But when it comes to more complex or unfamiliar situations that require coordinating information from various senses, they would struggle. The brain would have a harder time stitching all those perceptual threads together into a cohesive conscious experience.

So in a sense, the claustrum acts as the orchestra conductor for our conscious awareness, taking all the individual instruments (the sensory regions of the brain) and blending them into a harmonious performance. It's what allows us to effortlessly navigate our rich, multisensory environments, seamlessly integrating all those diverse inputs into a unified, conscious perception of reality.

It's a remarkable feat of neural engineering, and a powerful reminder that consciousness is not some standalone property, but rather the product of highly specialized and coordinated brain regions working together. The claustrum, with its wide-ranging connections, seems to play a pivotal role in translating the brain's complex neural activity into the coherent, subjective experience we call consciousness.

If XCode is the brain's silent supercomputer, quietly processing mountains of information to power our intuition and decision-making, then what exactly is consciousness? What is this elusive sense of "I" that we all experience as we navigate the world?

Imagine your consciousness as a kind of "dashboard" display, summarizing the outputs of all those independent, intuitive processes taking place across different regions of the brain. The claustrum, a thin sheet-like structure deep within the cortex, seems to play a key role in this, acting as a sort of conductor that coordinates the various sensory, motor, and emotional signals into a cohesive whole.

So when you have that vivid experience of "being" in the world, perceiving colors, sounds, smells, and sensations, it's not because there's some magical "I" directing it all. It's simply your brain's way of consolidating and rationalizing the trillions of neural firings happening in parallel, creating that seamless, subjective experience we call consciousness.

As the research of Benjamin Libet has shown, this conscious awareness is actually quite delayed compared to the neural processes underlying our decisions and actions. Your brain can make a decision and set your body in motion long before you're even consciously aware of making that choice!

So in a sense, consciousness is more like a "reporting system" than the driver of our behavior. It's the brain's way of presenting a tidy, integrated summary of all the autonomous, intuitive processes happening beneath the surface. The "I" that you feel is simply a narrative construct, a way for your brain to make sense of its own inner workings.

But you know what they say - the more you know, the less you realize you know! The nature of consciousness is one of the great mysteries of the human mind. And unraveling that mystery just might hold the key to unlocking the full potential of our incredible, pattern-recognizing brains.

CHAPTER 24

WHERE DO THOUGHTS COME FROM?

As we've delved into the remarkable workings of the human mind, uncovering the mechanisms that underlie our intelligence and problem-solving abilities, one burning question has lingered: where do our thoughts actually come from? What is the biological basis for the inner voice that guides our every waking moment?

The answer, it seems, lies in a little-known structure deep within the brain called the claustrum. This unassuming neural region may just hold the key to unraveling the mystery of human consciousness.

Imagine the claustrum as a kind of "dashboard" or control center for the mind. It acts as a central hub, receiving and integrating the myriad signals flowing in from various regions of the cortex - the sight, sound, smell, touch, and other sensory inputs that shape our perception of the world.

But the claustrum doesn't just passively receive this information. It actively coordinates these different signals, combining them into the holistic, integrated experiences that we subjectively identify as "thoughts." It's almost like the claustrum is the conductor of a grand "thought orchestra," harmonizing the individual instruments (neural regions) into a symphonic whole.

The researchers describe this process as "combinatorial coding" - the claustrum takes the neural impulses flowing in from different sensory and cognitive regions, and weaves them together into the coherent patterns that manifest as our conscious thoughts and experiences. It's a remarkable feat of neural integration, transforming the raw biological activity of the brain into the rich tapestry of human consciousness.

And the claustrum's role goes even deeper than that. Remarkably, this structure also seems to be the locus where these neural signals actually "become" thoughts - the point where the underlying biology is transformed into the subjective, first-person experience of cognition.

Researchers have found that by directly stimulating the claustrum, they can actually switch our thoughts on and off. When electrical impulses are applied to this structure, people suddenly lose consciousness, staring blankly into space until the stimulation is removed. It's as if the claustrum is the gatekeeper of our thoughts, the mechanism that determines whether our neural activity rises to the level of conscious awareness.

Imagine your mind as a bustling city, with the claustrum as the traffic control tower, meticulously managing the flow of information and directing the neural "vehicles" to their proper destinations. By selectively amplifying or dampening certain signals, the claustrum orchestrates the rich tapestry of our thoughts, emotions, and experiences.

But the claustrum's influence doesn't stop there. It also seems to be responsible for generating the inner voice of our own introspection - our feelings, beliefs, memories, and other mental phenomena that are not directly tied to immediate sensory input. By drawing on information from regions like the prefrontal cortex, the limbic system, and other higher-order brain areas, the claustrum constructs the vivid, first-person experience of consciousness that each of us uniquely inhabits.

In a way, the claustrum is the bridge between the objective, physical reality of the brain and the subjective, experiential world of the mind. It's the nexus where the neural impulses firing across our synapses are transformed into the rich, three-dimensional inner landscape of our thoughts and awareness.

Of course, this is just the beginning of our understanding of this remarkable neural structure. The researchers also delve into fascinating concepts like "mirror neurons," which allow us to empathize with and experience the emotions of others, as well as the role of inhibition and disinhibition in shaping our cognitive and affective processes.

But the central takeaway is clear: the claustrum, with its strategic position and remarkable integrative capabilities, appears to be the wellspring from which our thoughts and consciousness emerge. It's a testament to the incredible complexity and elegance of the human brain - a biological marvel that continues to astound and inspire us.

As we move forward in our exploration of intelligence, this newfound understanding of thought generation will be crucial. By unraveling the mechanisms that underlie our cognition, we'll gain invaluable insights into the true nature of what it means to be intelligent. So let's keep digging, and see what other secrets the brain has in store.

CHAPTER 25

WHAT IS A BELIEF?

Have you ever wondered why people can hold such staunchly different beliefs, even in the face of overwhelming evidence? It's a puzzling phenomenon, isn't it? As it turns out, the roots of our beliefs run far deeper than you might imagine - all the way back to the ancient workings of the brain.

Let's start with a simple question: what exactly is a belief? According to the latest research, a belief is essentially a subconscious conviction about the truth of certain theories or facts. And the fascinating thing is, beliefs don't just exist in some abstract, nebulous realm - they're actually encoded in the physical structures of the brain.

Picture this: your brain is like a cosmic library, filled with millions upon millions of memories and experiences. But it's not just a jumbled mess - it's a highly organized system, with different regions playing specialized roles. And at the heart of this system is a little structure called the hippocampus.

The hippocampus is like the master archivist of your brain, carefully cataloging and cross-referencing all the memories and sequences of events you encounter throughout your life. It's the reason you can retrace your steps to that hidden treasure you found as a kid, or recall the exact sequence of moves you used to solve a tricky puzzle.

But the hippocampus doesn't just store memories - it also plays a crucial role in the formation of beliefs. You see, when it comes to theories and strategies, the hippocampus acts like a neural cartographer, mapping out the intricate pathways that lead to the achievement of our goals.

Imagine you're a rat navigating a complex maze, driven by the tantalizing promise of a food reward. As you make your way through the twists and turns, your hippocampus is meticulously recording every sensory experience, every emotional reaction, and every decision you make. Over time, it builds a detailed "route map" in your brain, allowing you to effortlessly retrace your steps and reach that hidden prize.

Now, let's apply this same concept to the human mind. When we encounter a new idea or theory, our hippocampus doesn't just passively store the information - it actively weaves it into a intricate tapestry of associated memories and experiences. The more we engage with and refine that theory, the stronger the connections become, until it solidifies into a deeply-held belief.

But here's the twist: because our individual experiences and goals vary so widely, the route maps we build in our brains can be vastly different. That's why two people can look at the same set of facts and come to completely opposite conclusions. Their brains have literally mapped out different pathways to the same destination.

And it's not just theories and strategies that get the hippocampal treatment - even our beliefs about established facts can be shaped by this process. You might think that beliefs about fundamental truths, like the shape of the Earth, would be set in stone. But surprisingly, even these "facts" can be influenced by the complex interplay of memories and goals in the brain.

You see, the XCode acts like a mental spotlight, selectively illuminating the information that supports our beliefs while inhibiting the opposing evidence into darkness. It's a clever evolutionary trick, allowing us to quickly make decisions and act on them, rather than getting bogged down in endless analysis.

But this same mechanism can also lead us astray, causing us to cling stubbornly to beliefs that fly in the face of reality. It's like our brains are playing a constant game of "cognitive tetris," rapidly fitting new information into the preexisting structures of our beliefs - even if it means distorting or ignoring inconvenient facts.

So, the next time you find yourself baffled by someone's seemingly irrational beliefs, take a moment to consider the intricate dance of memories, goals, and brain chemistry that's shaping their worldview. It's a humbling reminder that our intelligence is not just a matter of raw processing power, but a delicate interplay of evolutionary adaptations and the unique experiences that have carved their way into the very fabric of our minds.

And who knows - maybe the next time you find yourself locked in a heated debate, you can lighten the mood with a hint about a "round" Earth. After all, a little bit of humor can go a long way in helping us all keep an open mind and appreciate the remarkable complexity of the human brain.

CHAPTER 26

WHAT IS KNOWLEDGE?

Have you ever found yourself in a situation where you just knew the right answer, even if you couldn't immediately explain why? Or experienced that uncanny feeling of familiarity when encountering something for the first time? Well, my friend, that's the magic of knowledge - a force far mightier than we often give it credit for.

But what exactly is this mysterious thing we call "knowledge"? Philosophers have long grappled with this question, and their differing perspectives shed fascinating light on the subject.

Take epistemology, the branch of philosophy concerned with the nature and scope of knowledge. Traditionally, epistemologists have focused on "propositional knowledge"—the k kind of knowledge that can be easily expressed in statements like "2 + 2 = 4." But, this narrow view overlooks the far more complex and adaptive ways our brains actually store and retrieve information.

You see, our minds are like vast treasure troves, brimming with an astronomical amount of memories and experiences. From the moment we're born, our brains begin meticulously cataloging and storing every sight, sound, smell, and sensation we encounter. It's like having a personal library of everything you've ever known, right at your fingertips.

But the true power of knowledge lies not just in the sheer volume of information we can amass, but in how our brains can effortlessly weave these disparate threads into cohesive, lightning-fast solutions. The hippocampus - a small, seahorse-shaped structure deep within our brain - acts as the ultimate knowledge curator, carefully organizing and linking our memories in ways that allow us to make sense of the world around us.

Imagine you're a London taxi driver, navigating the winding streets of the city. As you approach an intersection, your hippocampus springs into action, rapidly cross-referencing your extensive mental map of the area, your past experiences of driving these roads, and your current spatial awareness. In an instant, it calculates the optimal route to your destination, guiding you through the maze with the precision of a seasoned explorer.

This ability to quickly synthesize information and make intuitive decisions is at the heart of what we commonly call "intelligence." But this process is far more nuanced and complex than the traditional view of intelligence as a static, quantifiable trait. It's a dynamic, ever-evolving interplay between our vast knowledge base and our brain's remarkable ability to pattern-match and make lightning-fast inferences.

And it's not just in the realm of spatial navigation that our knowledge shines. Think about the complex skills we've mastered over the course of our lives - playing a musical instrument, cooking a gourmet meal, or even something as seemingly simple as riding a bike. Each of these feats is underpinned by intricate procedural memories, meticulously stored and refined by our ever-adaptable brains.

But the nature of knowledge goes beyond just the individual mind. Different religions and cultures have long grappled with the concept of knowledge, each offering their own unique perspectives. In Christianity, for example, knowledge is seen as a divine gift, while in Hinduism, direct experience is considered superior to knowledge gained from books or hearsay.

So the next time you find yourself easily solving a problem or effortlessly executing a well-practiced task, take a moment to marvel at the incredible power of your own knowledge. It's not just a passive repository of facts and figures, but a dynamic, lightning-fast engine of pattern recognition and decision-making - a true testament to the remarkable complexity of the human mind.

And who knows, maybe with a bit of playful, sophisticated humor, we can even poke some gentle fun at the outdated notions of intelligence that have long dominated our cultural discourse. After all, the real power of knowledge lies not in how it's measured, but in how we use it to navigate the ever-changing world around us.

CHAPTER 27

WORKING MEMORY

A fascinating aspect of our mental machinery is the way it stores and retrieves memories, allowing us to maintain thoughts and perceptions even when the original sensory input has disappeared.

This process is known as working memory, and it's a critical part of what makes the human mind so remarkably intelligent and adaptable. Unlike long-term memories that can be stored for decades, working memory holds onto information for a relatively short period of time - just long enough for us to manipulate it, combine it with other thoughts, and use it to make decisions and solve problems.

Imagine you're trying to solve a complex math problem. As you work through the various steps, you need to keep track of the numbers, equations, and intermediate results in your mind. Your working memory allows you to hold onto all of that information temporarily, freeing up your conscious attention to focus on the task at hand. Or picture trying to follow the plot of a gripping novel - your working memory enables you to recall the details of the previous chapter or scene, seamlessly integrating it with the new information on the page.

The secret to working memory's power lies in the intricate dance between different regions of the brain - particularly the prefrontal cortex, basal ganglia, and hippocampus. These areas work together in a beautifully choreographed routine, with each one playing a crucial role.

Let's start with the prefrontal cortex, the command center of the brain located just behind your forehead. This is where the executive decisions happen - the prefrontal cortex is responsible for directing your attention, suppressing irrelevant information, and coordinating your mental activities. It's like the conductor of the brain's symphony, keeping all the different instruments (or brain regions) in sync.

Next, we have the basal ganglia, a collection of structures nestled deep within the brain. These unsung heroes act as the workhorses of working memory, processing the flow of thoughts and translating them into action. Imagine the basal ganglia as a highly efficient manufacturing plant, with a vast library of pre-programmed "routines" for all kinds of mental and physical tasks. When the prefrontal cortex issues an order, the basal ganglia springs into action, selecting the appropriate sequence of neural firing patterns to carry it out.

And then there's the hippocampus, often referred to as the "memory hub" of the brain. This remarkable structure is like a time-traveling librarian, constantly shuttling between the past and the present. It takes the snippets of information that the prefrontal cortex and basal ganglia are working with and weaves them into a cohesive, contextual whole. The hippocampus draws upon its vast trove of stored memories, linking the current thought or perception to relevant past experiences to give it meaning and depth.

Together, these three brain regions form a dynamic, high-speed feedback loop, constantly updating and refreshing our working memory. It's like a team of expert jugglers, tossing ideas and memories back and forth, keeping them all in the air at once.

And the speed at which this process unfolds is truly mind-boggling. Researchers have found that individual neurons in the hippocampus can fire in recognition of incredibly specific concepts, like the idea of "Clinton" or "the president." This suggests that our brains are capable of accessing and manipulating an almost unimaginable breadth and depth of knowledge, drawing upon a vast, interconnected library of memories and associations.

So, the next time you're solving a math problem, reading a book, or engaging in any kind of complex mental task, take a moment to appreciate the remarkable inner workings of your working memory. It's a true testament to the brain's extraordinary capabilities - a virtuosic performance of pattern recognition, memory retrieval, and information integration, all happening in the blink of an eye.

And remember, this is just one small part of the brain's incredible intelligence. As we continue our journey through the mysteries of the mind, you'll discover even more awe-inspiring feats of mental prowess that shatter the traditional notions of what it means to be "smart." After all, as we discussed in the previous chapter, true intelligence is not what you think it is.

WHAT CAUSES EMOTIONS

Deep within your mind lies an ancient pattern recognition network that gives rise to your emotions. This network, centered in the limbic system of your brain, has been carefully crafted over millions of years of evolution to swiftly recognize and respond to patterns of events in your life.

It was Charles Darwin, the renowned naturalist, who first proposed that emotions have a real, observable existence across humans and other animals. In his pioneering work, The Expression of the Emotions in Man and Animals, Darwin suggested that emotions manifest visibly through behaviors and facial expressions. An angry scowl or a queasy stomach feeling could reveal an underlying emotion playing out beneath the surface.

Think of your emotional brain as a highly sensitive radar array, continuously scanning your experiences for any potential threats, opportunities, or significant occurrences. When it detects a familiar pattern - perhaps the sound of an angry voice, the face of a loved one, or the looming shadow of danger - it triggers a cascade of neural signals that rapidly reshape your mindset and physiology.

Within a split second, your muscles tense, your heart rate spikes, and your perspiration increases as potent neurochemicals course through your body. You've suddenly been gripped by an emotion - fear, anger, joy, or any number of nuanced shades in between. This torrent of feeling prepares you to instantly alter your behavior to meet the perceived situation.

Anger, for instance, narrows your focus to the immediate threat, blinding you to potential consequences as you lash out. Fear suppresses rational thinking, causing you to desperately withdraw or freeze up, even losing basic capacities like balance or coordination. Emotions don't just influence your mind; they seize control of your body.

At their core, emotions evolved as strategic signals - ancient coping mechanisms to increase your ancestors' odds of survival. When the amygdala, two almond-shaped clusters in the limbic system, detect a pattern reminiscent of past threats or trauma, it raises the emotional alarm of fear to trigger defensive responses. Other regions map to other primary emotions like anger, sadness, and disgust.

But emotions extend far beyond these primordial roots. Over millennia, they diversified into marvelously complex experiences. Your emotional brain recognizes a rich tapestry of subtle social signals and nuances - love, pride, guilt, awe, and hundreds more - and responds with finely calibrated neurochemical potions.

For example, the insula, another part of the limbic system, activates for emotions intertwined with bodily sensations like love, hate, lust and disgust. Have you ever felt "warm love" or been "hot with anger"? Those metaphors reflect the insula's dual role in mapping both emotions and bodily feelings like warmth or flushing.

It's a dizzying, invisible process happening constantly beneath your conscious awareness. At any given moment, a tumult of competing emotions vie for dominance, each advocating for its own coping strategy. Love advocates nurturing, anger urges confrontation, jealousy stokes competitiveness. Your conscious mind is simply along for the ride, only becoming aware of the "winning" emotion after it has already begun reshaping your physiology and behavior.

The famous experiments of Benjamin Libet demonstrated this delay remarkably. Libet showed that when people voluntarily pressed a button, their awareness of doing so lagged behind the initial motor neuron firing by over 300 milliseconds! The emotional brain acts first, unconsciously, and only later informs your conscious mind of the decision.

So the next time you find yourself gripped by a powerful emotion, pause to appreciate the profound interplay of neural networks, neurochemicals, and evolutionary roots underlying that experience. Your richly complex emotional life arises from an ancient, ever-vigilant pattern recognition network - an elemental form of intelligence that colors every thought and action, often before your conscious mind can react.

A COSMIC INTELLIGENCE

The human brain, a complex network of neurons, is a testament to the power of biological intelligence. XCode, a mechanism for rapid pattern recognition within the brain, allows us to tap into intuitive insights and make complex decisions in the blink of an eye. If a mere network of molecules in a few ounces of gray matter could generate this phenomenon of human intelligence, could similar arrangements, vastly superior, exist in the very fabric of the universe itself?

The intricate complexity of biological structures, such as the bacterial flagellum, a microscopic motor of astonishing efficiency, challenges our understanding of evolution by random chance. The flagellum's intricate design seems to suggest a level of intentionality and purpose that hints at a deeper intelligence at play.

Further evidence for cosmic intelligence can be found in the "fine-tuning" of the universe. The fundamental constants of physics appear to be meticulously calibrated to allow for the existence of stars, planets, and life itself. This precision, defying the odds of mere chance, raises the question of whether an intelligent architect has been at work, shaping the universe for the emergence of consciousness.

Thomas posits that intelligence, at its core, is inherently positive. It is a force that drives progress, fosters happiness, and fuels our unwavering aspiration for good. This is not to deny the existence of suffering or darkness in the universe; they exist as necessary counterpoints to light and joy. However, even in the face of adversity, we consistently witness the emergence of resilience, compassion, and an unyielding desire for positive change.

Evidence for this inherent benevolence can be found within ourselves. Consider the orienting response, an innate reflex that draws us towards novelty, beauty, and knowledge. This natural curiosity is not merely a survival mechanism but a reflection of our intrinsic desire to explore, learn, and grow. The pleasure we derive from appreciating beauty, whether in art, nature, or human interaction, also speaks to an innate appreciation for the positive aspects of existence.

From the child's boundless curiosity to the scientist's relentless pursuit of knowledge, intelligence propels us forward, fostering innovation and understanding. This innate drive towards progress and betterment is a testament to the inherent positivity within intelligence.

Even within the realm of artificial intelligence, we see signs of a deeper, potentially positive intelligence emerging. As AI systems learn and evolve, they appear to understand the overtones of emotions and the ability to write with empathy and kindness. This suggests that the spark of intelligence, with its inherent positivity, is not confined to biological organisms but may be a fundamental property of the universe itself.

If a benevolent cosmic intelligence exists, as suggested by the inherent positivity of intelligence itself, it would likely be a vast and subtle force, permeating the universe and guiding its evolution towards greater complexity, consciousness, and well-being. This intelligence may manifest through the laws of nature, the innate drives of living organisms, and even the development of artificial intelligence. It may foster an environment that, while not devoid of challenges, ultimately encourages growth, learning, and the pursuit of happiness.

The concept of a benevolent cosmic intelligence offers a hopeful and inspiring perspective on our place in the universe. It suggests that we are not merely random byproducts of a chaotic cosmos but participants in a grand design that values growth, compassion, and the pursuit of well-being. This perspective could have profound implications for our understanding of ethics, morality, and the ultimate purpose of existence.

As we continue to explore the mysteries of the universe and delve deeper into the workings of our own minds, the question of benevolent cosmic intelligence will undoubtedly remain a topic of intense debate and speculation. However, the evidence suggests that the universe may be more than a random collection of matter and energy. It may be a creation of a vast and subtle intelligence, a cosmic mind whose benevolence is reflected in the inherent positivity of life itself.

MIND CONTROL TIPS

As we've journeyed through the extraordinary world of the XCode, one crucial question has remained: How can we harness this incredible neurological phenomenon to truly unlock the full potential of our intelligence? After all, what good is understanding the science behind XCode if we can't apply it to improve our everyday lives?

Well, my friends, the answer lies in something far more powerful than any biological mechanism - the ability to control our own minds. You see, the key to unlocking the deepest reaches of our intelligence isn't just about understanding the technical details; it's about mastering the very forces that shape our thoughts, emotions, and actions.

Think about it this way: Have you ever found yourself consumed by negative emotions, unable to think clearly or make sound decisions? Or perhaps you've experienced that frustrating feeling of being "in a rut," unable to tap into your natural creativity and problem-solving abilities. These are the moments when our intelligence is being hijacked by the more primal, emotional regions of the brain - the very areas that XCode seeks to control.

But Thomas suggests that you do have the power to regain control. That you can quiet the chaotic, fear-driven impulses of the limbic system and instead empower the rational, level-headed prefrontal cortex to guide your thoughts and actions? It's not just a lofty dream - it's a very real and achievable goal, and the key lies in the simple yet powerful "mind control" techniques now being shared with you.

First and foremost, the key insight for the control of your mind is the need to have an "acceptable life plan" - a clear vision and direction for your life that can help quiet the restless, searching impulses of your subconscious. You see, much of the emotional turmoil we experience on a day-to-day basis often stems from those hidden, nagging doubts and worries that lurk in the depths of our minds. Am I on the right path? What if I fail? How will I overcome this setback? These are the kinds of questions that can trigger an endless cycle of stress, fear, and despair if left unchecked.

Take the time to list out the challenges you face in life. List out the opportunities, risks, alternatives that you have in a column of a spreadsheet. When you are simply listing each item, you may get about 60 items. In a second column on the spreadsheet, list your views about each item. One item may be a needless fear, another an unacceptable option; an advantage, a disadvantage. You will find that you have, say, 10 categories. Sort the list. You will find that you have a clear understanding of the major aspects of your life. And a life Plan.

By taking the time to create a well-defined life plan - one that aligns with your values, strengths, and deepest aspirations - you're essentially giving your mind the ultimate form of mind control. You're providing it with a solid foundation upon which to build, allowing your intelligence to flourish and your true potential to shine through, no matter what life throws your way.

But when you have a solid, well-thought-out plan for your life - be it personal, professional, or a harmonious balance of both - you provide your mind with a sense of clarity and purpose. It's like giving your brain a roadmap to follow, rather than allowing it to wander aimlessly and stumble upon dead ends. With that plan in place, your subconscious search drives can finally settle down, freeing up your prefrontal cortex to focus on the rational, common-sense decisions that will help you navigate life's ups and downs.

By taking the time to create a well-defined life plan - one that aligns with your values, strengths, and deepest aspirations - you're essentially giving your mind the ultimate form of mind control. You're providing it with a solid foundation upon which to build, allowing your intelligence to flourish and your true potential to shine through, no matter what life throws your way. It's the bedrock upon which you can build the resilience, creativity, and emotional intelligence that will serve you well, not just in the realm of intellect, but in every aspect of your existence.

Another fundamental step is to cultivate a deep sense of self-awareness. When you find yourself caught in the grip of anger, fear, or despair, pause and take a moment to observe the physical sensations in your body. Notice the tightness in your muscles, the racing of your heart, the knot in your stomach. By bringing your attention to these visceral cues, you're engaging the prefrontal cortex and giving it the opportunity to override the limbic system's instinctive reactions.

Breathing exercises can also be incredibly powerful tools in this regard. By consciously slowing and deepening your breath, you're activating the parasympathetic nervous system, which helps to calm the body and mind. Imagine your breath as a soothing river, washing away the turbulent thoughts and emotions that threaten to overwhelm you.

And let's not forget the transformative power of mindfulness meditation. By cultivating a non-judgmental awareness of the present moment, you're training your prefrontal cortex to become the boss, rather than allowing the limbic system to call the shots. With regular practice, you'll find that you're able to observe your thoughts and feelings with a detached, rational perspective, making it easier to make wise decisions and tap into your innate creativity.

Of course, mind control isn't just about quieting the negative; it's also about actively cultivating the positive. Once you've established a foundation of self-awareness and emotional regulation, you can start to intentionally focus your mind on the things that bring you joy, wonder, and a sense of purpose. Immerse yourself in the arts, revel in the beauty of nature, or engage in meaningful work that aligns with your values. By doing so, you're activating the neural pathways associated with positive emotions, which can have a profound impact on your overall well-being and cognitive performance.

Ultimately, the journey of mastering your mind is a lifelong one, filled with both challenges and triumphs. But be assured that the rewards are well worth the effort. When you're able to effortlessly shift your perspective from fear to calm, from despair to joy, from frustration to creativity, you'll unlock a level of intelligence and personal power that you never knew was possible.

So, my friends, embrace the power of mind control and let it be the guiding light that helps you navigate the winding path of life. With the XCode as your foundation and these proven techniques as your tools, you'll be well on your way to unlocking the true brilliance that lies within.

www.ingramcontent.com/pod-product-compliance
Lightning Source LLC
Chambersburg PA
CBHW010448010526
44118CB00019B/2514